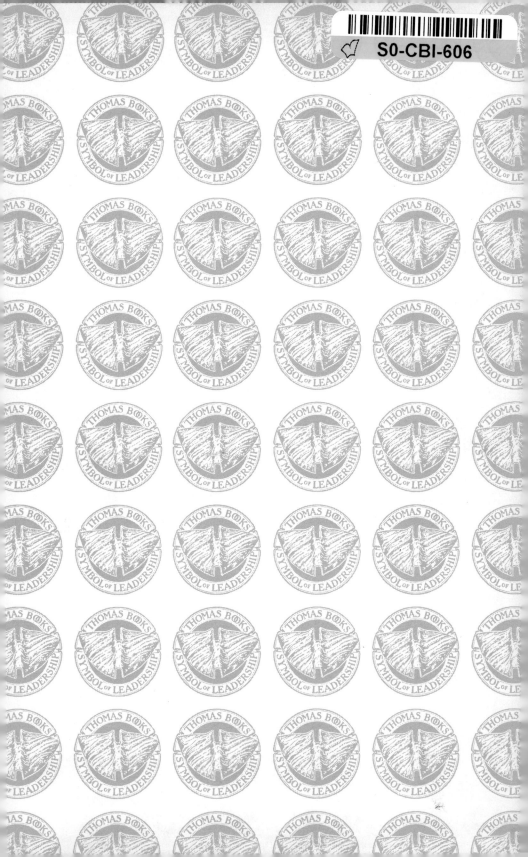

CORONARY ANGIOGRAPHY

CORONARY ANGIOGRAPHY

By

HAROLD A. BALTAXE, M.D.

Associate Professor of Radiology
Cornell Medical College
Head, Division of Cardiovascular Radiology
New York Hospital
New York, New York

KURT AMPLATZ, M.D.

Professor of Radiology
University of Minnesota Medical School
Chief, Cardiovascular Radiology
University of Minnesota Hospital
Minneapolis, Minnesota

DAVID C. LEVIN, M.D.

Assistant Professor of Radiology
Cornell Medical College
New York, New York

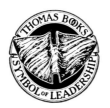

CHARLES C THOMAS • PUBLISHER
Springfield • Illinois • U.S.A.

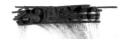

Published and Distributed Throughout the World by
CHARLES C THOMAS • PUBLISHER
BANNERSTONE HOUSE
301-327 East Lawrence Avenue, Springfield, Illinois, U.S.A.

© *1973, by* CHARLES C THOMAS • PUBLISHER

ISBN 0–398–02709–9

Library of Congress Catalog Card Number: 72–88439

Printed in the United States of America

BB-14

This book is dedicated to
THEM

PREFACE

Coronary artery disease is the prime killer of middle-aged and older men and women. As time has passed, we have discovered that even younger individuals are not spared by this disease. For years surgeons have tried to provide a remedy for angina caused by coronary arteriosclerosis, and for years they have failed. What could be simpler than to bypass a stenotic segment of a vessel and to restore adequate perfusion distal to the narrowing? In fact, it is very difficult! Lately, however, new surgical procedures have come into being, and they seem to hold some promise. Whatever the surgical approach might be, today or tomorrow, it is obvious that precise anatomic representation of the coronary arteries will always be necessary to plan adequate surgical and sometimes medical therapy.

For decades clinicians tried to visualize the coronary arteries, and yet coronary angiography only became available in the sixties. Today the feasibility of coronary angiography is not questioned anymore. What might be questioned is, How many procedures can one perform each day?

We have attempted in this book to help clinicians involved in the diagnosis and treatment of coronary artery disease to interpret coronary angiograms. We could have discussed some sections in this book in greater depth, but our main concern was to remain practical! This book is far from being an encyclopedia, but perhaps it will be a guide.

We have emphasized the number of illustrations, believing that one good picture is better than many words. We hope that as radiologists we have not been too biased and that this work will not be directed only to members of our specialty.

I wanted to begin this preface with "I once had a dream," but that has been said before! Therefore, I will restrict myself to saying that the idea for this book was conceived in the fall of 1969 and that it took a long time to realize "my dream." The time spent was not all devoted to work—we had fun writing this book, but foremost, we learned a lot doing it! Since I am taking the liberty of writing this preface, I want to emphasize that without the guidance and invaluable help of my co-authors, this book would never have been written.

All three of us sincerely hope that this book will help the reader in his or her studies and practice.

HAROLD A. BALTAXE

ACKNOWLEDGMENTS

We are grateful and indebted to everyone who was involved in the making of this book.

At New York Hospital, we wish to thank Dr. John Evans for his continuous support. Special thanks are also due to the members of the Department of Surgery (Drs. Ebert, C.W. Lillehei, Carlson, Gay, and Block) and to the members of the Department of Cardiology (Drs. Killip, Rosenfeld, Ettinger, Scheidt, Winston, Nydick, Pritchett, and many others) who have been kind enough to entrust their patients to our care. For the excellent technical help we are indebted to our x-ray technicians and to our marvelous nurses. The drawings were done by Lynn McDowell who showed great dedication. Photography was performed by the staff of the Department of Medical Photography who have been relentless in their cooperation. We also wish to thank our secretaries in the Division of Cardiovascular Radiology at New York Hospital. Two left us in the process, but Mrs. Dorothy Miller, who has the incomparable talent to read H.A.B.'s handwriting, deserves special thanks. Without her help, it would have taken us another three years to finish this book.

At the University of Minnesota, we wish to thank Drs. Peterson and Gedgaudas for their support during H.A.B.'s stay in their department. Special thanks to the technicians in the Heart Hospital.

We are indebted to Squibb Laboratories for their financial support which allowed us initially to get started with our project.

Finally, many thanks to the students, residents, and fellows for stimulating us and reminding us that our prime goal should be to teach.

CONTENTS

xi

CORONARY ANGIOGRAPHY

CHAPTER I

HISTORY OF CORONARY ANGIOGRAPHY

The injection of a radiopaque substance into the vessel of a live patient was first performed by Egas Moniz in 1927.[1] Three years later Dos Santos, Lamas, and Caldas performed the first abdominal aortogram. It is, however, Forssman who became the Father of Selective Angiography by introducing in 1929 a rubber catheter from the left cephalic vein into the right atrium of his heart.[2] Only four years later Rousthoi utilized Forssman's technique to opacify the coronary artery tree.[3] He performed a cut down on the right carotid artery of a rabbit and introduced a catheter into the ascending aorta just above the aortic valve, through which he injected a contrast material. These early radiographs demonstrated the coronary arteries with amazingly good detail. In 1933, Reboul described a method of right and left ventriculography by a direct percutaneous ventricular puncture in the animals, injecting the contrast medium through the needle.[4] One of his greatest contributions, however, was in realizing that serial films were necessary and he advocated obtaining several exposures at the time of injection (from two to six radiographs in ten to thirty seconds). Apparently from 1933 till 1945 no one showed great interest in the visualization of the coronary arteries. Radner in 1945 revived the subject with his "Attempt at the Roentgenologic Visualization of the Coronary Blood Vessels in Man."[5] Today, his method would appear somewhat cruel; however, it took courage to implement such a technique! The patient was in the sitting position while a needle was introduced percutaneously into the ascending aorta. The needle tip was placed just above the aortic valve and Thorotrast was injected into the aorta resulting in the opacification of the ascending aorta and the coronary arteries.

In the fifties, with the advent of Seldinger's percutaneous

catheterization technique, selective angiography became a widely accepted diagnostic tool. Nonetheless, most investigators were reluctant to introduce the catheter tip directly into the ostium of the coronary arteries. Thus, many nonselective and semi-selective techniques were developed. Since most of them have nothing but historical value, only a few of them will be described in this chapter.

In the early days of coronary angiography, the rapid delivery of a large bolus of contrast medium into the root of the aorta was the most widely utilized method of coronary angiography. As early as 1952, Di Guglielmo[6A-B] reported his experience with the examination of 235 patients with 112 satisfactory coronary artery visualizations. With the development of pressure injectors allowing a more rapid delivery of contrast material, and the utilization of large bore catheters (9F and 10F), better angiograms were obtained. One of the major technical difficulties, however, remained the delivery of contrast medium near to the coronary ostia in sufficiently high concentration in order to allow visualization of the diseased small coronary arterial tree. During each systole, the deposited contrast medium tended to be washed away and the opaque injected during diastole was lost and markedly diluted. Satisfactory opacification of the coronary arteries proved particularly difficult in patients with coronary artery disease due to the much smaller caliber of the diseased arteries and the slow and decreased coronary flow. The use of end occluded catheters with numerous side holes was helpful in delivering the contrast medium against the wall of the aorta. These catheters could also be more precisely positioned at the level of the coronary ostia since there was little if any recoil phenomenon.

In 1957 Dotter introduced a balloon catheter through the radial artery of a dog and placed it a few centimeters above the aortic valve.[7] The balloon was inflated with nitrous oxide or carbon dioxide and complete occlusion of the aorta was obtained for five to ten seconds while 5 ml of contrast was injected proximal to the balloon. This method was subsequently utilized in man but was not without complications.

Also in 1957, Arnulf in France[8] made the incidental discovery that the coronary arteries were beautifully opacified in an animal suffering from cardiac arrest. He subsequently induced cardiac arrest by the intravenous injection of acetylcholine and performed coronary arteriography in three hundred animals. This technique proved to be simple and resulted in reliable excellent visualization of the coronary arteries. The cardiac arrest lasting several seconds could be terminated by the intravenous injection of atropine or by cardiac massage. Three milligrams per kilogram of body weight of acetylcholine in saline were injected intravenously, producing cardiac arrest, at which time 15 ml of opaque medium were injected rapidly through an end occluded needle which had been introduced into the ascending aorta via suprasternal aortic puncture. Biplane angiographic studies were obtained at six exposures per second.

This technique was later modified and the contrast material was injected through a catheter. It was widely used in Europe as well as in some institutions in the United States. The excellent results obtained in animals could not be reproduced in humans. The main coronary arteries tended to be opacified but their peripheral ramifications were no longer filled, giving the wrong impression of coronary artery occlusion. Furthermore, contrast filling was largely dependent upon gravity thus demonstrating the left coronary artery better than the right coronary in the supine position.

Since coronary flow occurs predominently during diastole, diastolic dye injection was advocated by Richards,[9] at the University of Minnesota, who described in 1958 a compressed nitrogen driven syringe and an electronic dye injection control system, triggered by the R wave of the electrocardiogram. He introduced a closed-tip catheter 1 cm above the aortic valve and performed an injection of contrast material that extended from the onset of diastole to the conclusion of diastole. The injection time was from 0.2 to 1.6 seconds while biplane films were obtained at 5 exposures per second. The results were better than with nonphasic techniques. However, as with all nonselective methods, no peripheral filling of the coronary arteries was obtained.

Bellman *et al.*[10] in 1960 developed a loop polyethylene cathe-

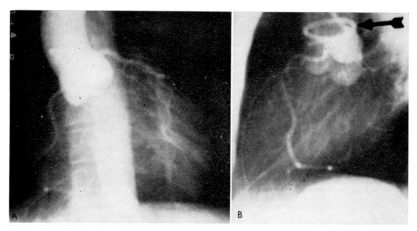

Figure 1. A, Anteroposterior view of a coronary arteriogram performed with a loop catheter. B, Lateral view. Arrow points to the loop.

ter with three side holes. This catheter was placed into the aortic root in such a fashion that two of the side holes lay opposite the coronary ostia regardless of catheter rotation. This catheter was better known as the Littman Williams catheter which was introduced over a flexible guide wire into the surgically exposed carotid or femoral artery. The results were excellent when the radiographic exposure was triggered by the EKG.

Later, this catheter was modified by others resulting in a corkscrew shape with numerous lateral side holes delivering the contrast medium in high concentration laterally against the aortic wall beyond the confine of a systolic stream (Fig. 1). Consequently there was very little dilution of contrast medium and opacification of the coronary arteries was excellent. One of the drawbacks of this most elegant semi-selective technique was difficulty in positioning of the catheter, which tended to be encompassed by the aortic valve leaflets during systole and pulled into the ventricle during diastole. Since this catheter slipped so easily through the aortic valve it was later used for left ventriculography.

Simpler means of decreasing cardiac output were implemented. Nordenstrom[11] advocated elevation of the intra-bronchial pressure to about 25 cm of water resulting in a drop of the systemic pressure to about 70 mm Hg and marked decrease of systemic flow. Two catheters were introduced by way of bilateral percutaneous transfemoral approaches. A very thin polyethylene catheter was placed into the femoral artery to monitor the systemic pressure and a large one into the ascending aorta for the injection of contrast medium (1 cc/kg of 76% methylglucamine diatrizoate). Nordenstrom also emphasized the importance of gravity, placing the coronary arteries into a dependent position by having the patient sit in front of a biplane changer. Excellent films were obtained but the method was cumbersome.

In 1964, Bilgutay *et al.*[12] introduced a venous pacemaker into the right atrium and by increasing the cardiac rate decreased the cardiac output. Injections of contrast into the root of the aorta were performed under those conditions. The method had the same disadvantages as all other nonselective methods (Fig. 2).

Sones, in 1959, introduced a selective technique which revolutionized coronary angiography. At the eighth annual convention of the American College of Cardiology in Philadelphia, he

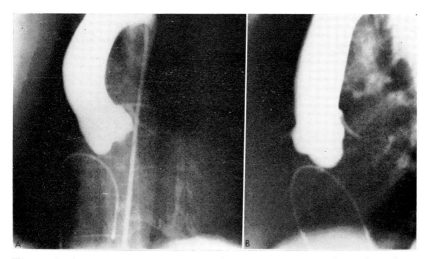

Figure 2. A, Anteroposterior view of an aortogram performed with a venous pacemaker in the right atrium. B, Lateral view. In spite of induced tachycardia the coronary arteries are poorly visualized.

described a method for selectively visualizing the coronary arteries.[13] Initially, in October of 1958, he had made deliberate attempts to perform "selective" coronary arteriography. Serial injections of 20 cc to 30 cc of contrast media were slowly introduced over a period of three to six seconds, directly into the right and left anterior sinuses of Valsalva.[14] Then, in April 1959, he designed a special catheter which permitted direct catheterization of the human coronary arteries. Thus, his contribution was to prove to the medical world that one could safely inject a contrast agent directly into the coronary ostia.

Since then, different techniques of selective coronary arteriography have been developed. In 1962, Ricketts and Abrams[15] described the first percutaneous transfemoral approach. Both the Sones' and percutaneous transfemoral methods have become widely used in recent years and will be discussed in detail in following chapters.

REFERENCES

1. Moniz, E., DeCarvalho, L., and Lima, A.: Angiopneumographie. *Presse Med.*, 39:996, 1931.
2. Forssman, W.: Die Sondierung des Rechten Herzens. *Klin Wochenschr*, 45:2085–87, Nov. 1929.
3. Rousthoi, P.: Ueber Angiokardiographie Vorlanfige Mitteilung.
4. Reboul, H., and Racine, M.: La Ventriculographie Cardiaque Experimentale. *Presse Med.*, 1:763, 1933.
5. Radner, S.: An attempt at the roentgenologic visualization of the coronary blood vessels in man. *Acta Radiol.* 26:497, 1945.
6A. DiGuglielmo, L., and Guttaduro, M.: Roentgenologic study of coronary arteries in living. *Acta Radiol. (Stockh.), Suppl. 97*, Dec. 1952.
6B. DiGuglielmo L., and Guttaduro, M.: Visualization of arteries in living; review of 413 observations. *Radiol. Med.*, 40:945–975, Oct. 1954.
7. Dotter, C.T., and Frische, L.H.: Visualization of the coronary circulation by occlusion aortography: a practical method. *Radiology*, 76:502, 1958.
8. Arnulf G., and Chacornac, R.: Communication to La Societe de Chirurgie de Lyon, Nov. 14, 1957.
   Arnulf, G.: L'Arteriographie Methodique des Arteres Coronaires Grace a L'Utilisation de L'Acetylcholine. Donnees Experimentales et Cliniques. *Bull. Acad. Nat. Med.*, 25–26:661–71, 1958.

9. Richards, L.S., and Thal, A.P.: Phasic dye injection control system for coronary arteriography in the human. *Surg. Gynec. Obst., 107:* 739, 1958.

10. Bellman, S., Frank H.A., Lambert, P.B., Littman, D., and Williams, J.A.: Coronary arteriography. I. Differential opacification of the aortic stream catheters of special design-experimental development. *New Engl J. Med., 262:*325, 1960.

11. Nordenstrom,, B.: Contrast examination of the cardiovascular system during increased intrabronchial pressure. *Acta Radiol., Supp. 200,* 110 pp., 1960.

12. Bilgutay, A.M., Gannon, P., Sterns, L.P., Ferlic, R., and Lillehei, C.W.: Coronary arteriography. New method under induced hypotension by pacing-experimental and clinical application. *Arch. Surg., 89/5:* 899–904, 1964.

13. Sones, F.M. Jr.: Coronary Arteriography. Read before the 8th Annual Convention of the American College of Cardiology, Philadelphia, 1959.

14. Sones, F.M., Jr., *et al.:* Cine coronary arteriography. In Abstracts of 32nd Scientific Sessions of American Heart Assoc. *Circulation, 20:* 773, Oct. 1959.

15. Ricketts, H.J., and Abrams, H.L.: Percutaneous selective coronary cine arteriography. *J.A.M.A., 181:*620–624, 1962.

CHAPTER II

TECHNIQUES OF SELECTIVE CORONARY ANGIOGRAPHY—SONES TECHNIQUE

This represents the first technique of selective coronary angiography[1] and probably the most widely used approach amongst cardiologists. It is a very safe technique, and by 1970 Sones had performed over 20,000 studies.

To selectively catheterize the coronary arteries, Sones developed a catheter made of woven Dacron (manufactured by U.S. Catheters and Instruments Corp.) (see Fig. 3). Two types of catheters are available. Type I has a tip length of 1.5 inches whereas Type II has a 1 inch length. All the catheters have a 7 French lumen tapered to a 5.5F tip. Two outer diameters are available (7F and 8F) but both have a 7F lumen; thus, the 8F has a heavier wall. Four side holes are near the tip. Different catheter lengths are available. A "Positrol" coronary catheter is also manufactured; it has a fine stainless steel wire mesh incorporated in the wall which results in greater torque control.

Preoperatively, the patient is prepared in the following manner:

1. NPO after breakfast.
2. CR BICILLIN 1.2M units.
3. NA PHENOBARBITAL 200 mg intramuscularly.

The procedure is done under electrocardiographic control and constant arterial pressure monitoring, with an intravenous drip of a 5% G-W and Heparin running. Defibrillating equipment is readily available.

The patient is placed on a Cordis rotating cradle which is manipulated by the operator with a sterilized electrical handle. The technique consists of introducing the catheter through a

10

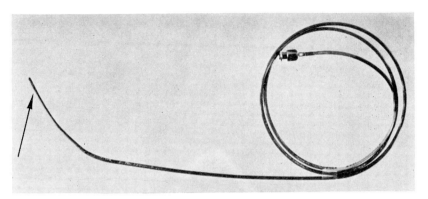

Figure 3. Sones catheter used for selective coronary angiography. Note that there are side holes (arrow) making ventriculography possible.

right brachial artery cut down into the ascending aorta. Under fluoroscopic control the catheter is then placed selectively into the right and left coronary arteries. The selective catheterization of the right coronary artery by this technique is relatively easy. The patient is turned into a left anterior oblique and the catheter is advanced from the ascending aorta to the ostium of the right coronary artery, in such a manner that the mild curve of the catheter is turned to the patient's right. A direct entry into the ostium is made, and thus one must take care to prevent occlusion of the vessel by the catheter. The constant pressure monitoring detects occlusion of the vessel by the catheter when damping of the pressure tracing occurs. Once the catheter is selectively in place, a small test dose of contrast is injected and results in visualization of the coronary artery. When the placement of the catheter is satisfactory 3 to 6 cc of a solution of Hypaque 90 diluted to 69% are injected by hand and cineangiography is obtained in several obliquities.* Multiple views are taken between 5 degrees to 20 degrees right anterior oblique, and 40 degrees to 60 degrees left anterior oblique.

The left coronary artery is often more difficult to catheterize. The same catheter is used. Without preshaped catheters a direct

---

* This is a description of the original technique. Dr. Sones now uses Renografin 76 instead of Hypaque 69%.

entry into the left coronary ostium is impossible and therefore the operator must shape the catheter inside the ascending aorta. Usually the catheter is pressed against the bottom of the aortic sinus in order to obtain a J shape. Once the shape is available the tip is directed slightly posteriorly and cephalad towards the ostium of the coronary artery. It is not unusual for the catheter to hit the roof of the vessel rather than to enter the vessel itself. However, this position is adequate for good opacification. Again, cineangiography is obtained in both oblique projections.

Selective coronary angiograms are always preceded by a left ventriculogram, which is performed with the same Sones catheter. This study is also recorded on 35 mm motion picture film, with the patient in the right anterior oblique projection.* If a revascularization procedure is contemplated, the assessment of the ventricular function and the identification of areas of scarring are of prime importance.

Coronary angiography performed by this method requires skill and excellent radiographic equipment. Sones very emphatically recommends the following type of equipment:

1. The generator should be full wave rectified and have a 500 mA and 150 kv capacity.
2. The x-ray table should be a free floating table top with 50 inch longitudinal movement equipped with electromagnetic brakes. There is to be a motor driven patient rotator with 60 degree rotation to either side.
3. The tube should be a high speed (8,500 rpm) rotating anode tube with 0.6 by 0.6 and 1.2 by 1.2 mm effective focal spots. During fluroscopy the anode should be stationary and for cineradiography the anode should be accelerated to high speed in 0.8 seconds. The tube capacity is to be 150 kw.
4. The intensifier is to have a 6 inch diameter input screen. The resolution is to be 50 lined pairs per inch centrally, and 30 lined pairs per inch peripherally.† Minimal visible contrast is to be 4%.

---

* Of late a second injection in the left anterior oblique projection has been added.

† Since these specifications were written, more sophisticated image amplifiers and x-ray tubes have appeared on the market.

5. The motion picture camera should be a 35 mm Arriflex camera with magazine and pulsing contact. The film frame rate should continuously be variable from 22 to 80 frames per second.

It is recommended that all equipment except the movie camera should be of the same manufacturer to insure perfect integration.

It is advised that the following ancillary equipment be available:

1. An automatic processor with temperature control which processes film at four feet per minute.*
2. A 35 mm projector viewer with rotating prism, counter and speed control and no threading required. Kodak XX 35 mm film is to be used; according to Sones it seems to be the best choice insofar as speed, graininess, detail, and contrast are concerned.

The usual surgical pack and instruments are used and will not be described here. Worthy of description is a manifold shown in Figure 4.† This manifold permits the connection of the catheter to a pressure recorder as well as to the contrast material and the heparinized solution of 5% glucose and water.

In conclusion this very precise technique has been used successfully by many operators. The possible criticisms are the following:

1. The necessity of an arterial cut down which is technically more difficult than the percutaneous technique, and presumes that the operator has mastered a vascular surgical technique which allows him to repair the arteriotomy.
2. Although it has been said that thrombosis of the brachial artery is of no consequence and should not be operated upon,[2] we have seen many patients with severe complaints, due to occlusion of this vessel.

---

* Sones recommends a Fisher Mark 16/35 processor using Hunt Cine developer and Flast-O-Graph-Fixer at a speed of 25 ft/min.
† Manufactured by Becton, Dickinson and Co., Rutherford, New Jersey.

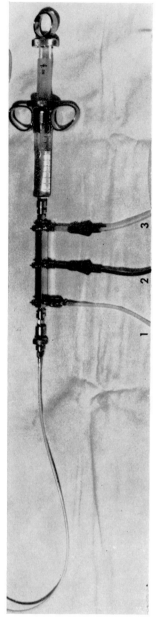

Figure 4. Manifold as used by Sones and now adopted by us. 1) Connecting tube going to the pressure transducer. 2) Contrast. 3) Flushing solution.

3. The catheter cannot always be selectively introduced into the lumen of the left coronary artery which may result in unsatisfactory opacification.
4. The technique is more difficult to learn than the ones which will be described in the next chapter.

REFERENCES

1. Sones, F.M. Jr., and Shirey, E.K.: Cine Coronary Arteriography, Modern Concepts of Cardiovascular Disease Vol. XXXI, No. 7, July 1962.
2. Sones, F.M. Jr.: Personal communication.

CHAPTER III

TECHNIQUES OF SELECTIVE CORONARY ANGIOGRAPHY—PERCUTANEOUS SELECTIVE CORONARY ARTERIOGRAPHY

In 1962, three years after Sones described his technique, Ricketts and Abrams developed a percutaneous approach to coronary arteriography.[1] Their contribution consisted of introducing preshaped catheters percutaneously from the femoral artery. They also found that a different shaped catheter was needed for each coronary artery. The material used was polyethylene tubing curved in near boiling water to conform to the aortic arch with the tip pointing towards either the right or left coronary ostium. The radius of the curvature of the right coronary catheter was made greater than that of the aortic arch, so that the tip tended to spring against the right anterior wall of the ascending aorta, thus facilitating cannulation of the right coronary ostium. The aortic arch curve of the left coronary catheter was continued dorsally, forming a complete circle, so that the tip extended to follow the left posterior wall of the ascending aorta. Side holes were not used, because they tended to weaken the tip of the catheter and diminished the reliability when monitoring the pressure.

Subsequently, Amplatz et al.[2] tested many commercially available materials for curvature memory and transmission of torque. They demonstrated that virgin radiopaque polyethylene showed the best memory. Polyurethane was slightly inferior, but Teflon and woven Dacron were extremely poor in retaining their shapes. The best transmission of torque was accomplished with woven Dacron of the "Positrol" design,*

* Manufactured by United States Catheter and Instrument Corp., Box 787, Glens Falls, New York.

16

followed closely by polyurethane with incorporated wire mesh. Although poor, Teflon was superior to polyethylene. The polyurethane catheters with incorporated wire mesh are now produced by the Cordis Corporation under the trade name of Ducor catheters. Using that catheter material Wilson *et al.*[3] and Judkins[4] developed two separate sets of coronary catheters, both of which are now commonly used and commercially available.*

THE AMPLATZ TECHNIQUE

In 1963 Amplatz described a technique for percutaneous infraclavicular catheterization of the right subclavian artery[5] which was used for coronary arteriography. Polyethylene catheters similar to the configuration described by Sones were used. Entry into the right coronary ostium was found to be relatively easy by this approach but selective catheterization of the left coronary ostium was more difficult. Because of occasional difficulties in puncturing the subclavian artery and problems with hemostasis following the withdrawal of the catheter, this approach was abandoned.

Since 1966, a percutaneous transfemoral catheterization technique has been successfully used at the University of Minnesota Hospitals which was described in detail in 1967 by Wilson *et al.*[3]

Catheterization of the *left coronary artery* is performed with the catheter shaped as shown in Figure 5L. This catheter has an outer diameter of 8 F and is available in four sizes, depending on the size and shape of the ascending aorta and aortic sinuses which are estimated from a chest roentgenograph. Particularly in males, with uncoiling of the ascending aorta, a size #3 will be successful; in females and younger patients size #2 will be adequate. Catheter size #1 is only used in very young patients and sometimes in females with small aortas as seen in congenital and rheumatic heart disease. On some occasions, a selective catheter may be too large or too small which is readily recognized during fluoroscopy, and requires

* Manufactured by the Cordis Corporation, Miami, Florida.

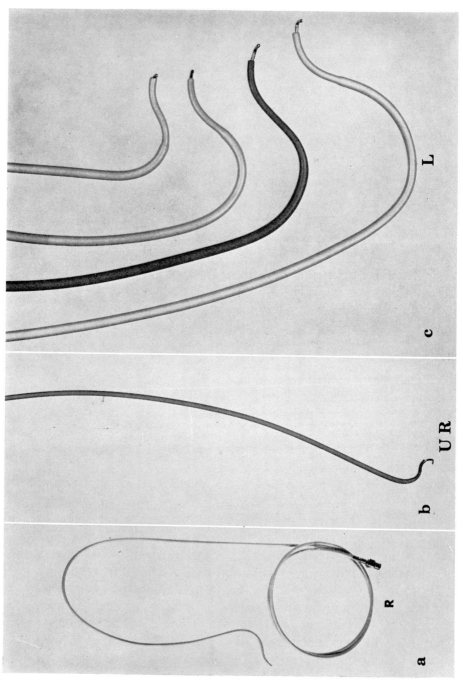

Figure 5. Right (R and UR) and left (L) selective coronary catheters as described by Amplatz, a, R—Conventional Right Coronary Catheter (available in 3 sizes). b, UR—Universal Right Catheter—Developed after the conventional right catheter and only available in one size. c, L—Left Coronary Catheters (available as shown here in 4 sizes).

catheter exchange. No time should be wasted with a catheter which is not of the proper size. With the proper catheter, intubation of the left coronary artery can even be performed by the novice. The left catheter has a J-shaped curve which is forcefully braced against the aortic valve (see Fig. 6 L^a). This causes a gradual upward motion of the catheter tip towards the ostium of the left coronary artery. The terminal curve near the tip of the catheter has a smaller diameter (5 F) and a slight countercurve preventing antegrade advancement of the catheter and mechanical obstruction of the coronary artery. Under fluoroscopy, using small test injections, it is determined how far the catheter tip has entered the coronary ostium. If the patient has a short main coronary artery or the catheter tip lies too close to the bifurcation of the anterior descending and left circumflex arteries, further pressure of the catheter against the aortic valve causes a retraction of the catheter tip back into the aorta. This mechanism is demonstrated for the right catheter (but also applies for the left) in Figure 6 R^a and R^b. On the other hand, by pulling the catheter gently back, its tip will further advance into the coronary artery (see Fig. 6 L^a and L^b). For most patients these adjustments are not necessary. Once the catheter is correctly positioned, it is not easily dislodged and the patient can be moved into various positions during angiography.

Inability to catheterize the left coronary artery may be due to too large or too small a catheter, or its lying anterior or posterior to the coronary ostium. Under those circumstances, proper rotation of the catheter may lead to success.

The *right coronary artery catheter* is available in three sizes, but the smallest shape is adequate for almost all patients. The shape of the catheter is identical to the left, but in addition a gentle, reversed curve conforming to the aortic arch facilitates rotation anteriorly in the direction of the right coronary artery (see Fig. 5 R). Under fluoroscopic control, the catheter is advanced into the ascending aorta. Sometimes manipulation at the level of the arch is necessary to prevent entry into the brachiocephalic vessels. Very uncommonly a guidewire has to be used in order to reach the ascending aorta. Fluoroscopy is

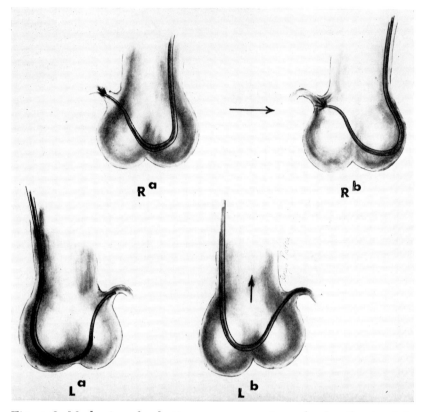

Figure 6. Mechanics of selective coronary angiography by the Amplatz method. R Catheterization of the Right orifice. Note that if the catheter is pushed the tip does not advance into the coronary artery but falls into the aorta (R^b). L^a Catheterization of the left ostium. As the catheter is pulled back (see arrow), the tip advances into the coronary artery (L^b).

performed in the supine position. In this position, the catheter tip should point straight anteriorly in order to enter the right coronary artery which is projected over the mid portion of the coronary sinus.

Recently a "universal" right coronary catheter, available in one size only, has been developed (see Fig. 6 UR). With this catheter, a direct entry is possible.

For direct right coronary artery catheterization with the universal right catheter, it is important that the catheter tip not be braced against the aortic valve since this impairs rotation. The catheter tip should be slightly above the aortic valve at the expected level of the coronary ostium, thus facilitating free rotation. At all times rotation should be combined with a simultaneous small backward or forward motion facilitating catheter control. Only the conventional right catheters can be introduced indirectly by bracing against the aortic cusp.

If the conventional right catheters are used, their size has to be matched to the size of the aorta. When the catheter is too large, its tip tends to be trapped in the aortic sinus and the curve cannot be reconstituted (see Fig. 7A). Increasing pressure against the aortic cusp as used for left coronary catheterization may cause the catheter to migrate above the right coronary ostium (see Fig. 7B). Figure 7 demonstrates the failure to catheterize the left coronary artery, but the same mechanism applies for the right.

Premedication

The following premedications have proved useful but may be altered depending on patient's age, psychologic status, etc.:

1. NPO after midnight.
2. Basic sedation of choice, commonly barbiturates and antihistamines (100 mg Seconal and 50 mg to 100 mg Visteril IM on call).
3. Additional sedatives such as Valium may be added or replace the above mentioned basic sedation.
4. An intravenous infusion of 5% glucose is started on call to the laboratory.

Atropine may be given as a premedication in order to minimize a hypotensive reaction. If coronary arteriograms are recorded on radiographic film, the tachycardia introduced by Atropine is undesirable; and, consequently, it is not administered routinely.

Procedure

Following percutaneous puncture of the femoral artery, a #8 ventriculography catheter is introduced into the left ventri-

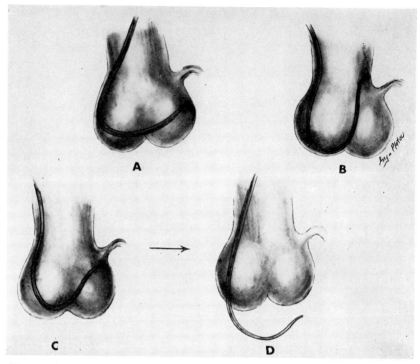

Figure 7. Demonstration of failure of catheterizing the left coronary artery because of inadequate catheter size. Amplatz method. A, Catheter is too big and trapped in the sinus. B, Catheter doubled up but reaches too high. C, Catheter is too small and does not reach the orifice. D, When the same catheter (C) is pushed to make it reach the ostium, it falls into the left ventricle. The same mechanism applies for the right coronary artery catheterization.

cle and ventricular pressures are recorded. A cine left ventriculogram is performed in the left posterior oblique position at a frame rate of sixty exposures per second. If left ventricular function appears abnormal as seen on the television screen, an additional injection of 50 cc of 76% diatrizoate contrast medium is made in the left anterior oblique position. The target film distance is kept constant in order to standardize magnification factors important for computation of physiologic parameters from the cine left ventriculogram.

From the cine left ventriculogram the left ventricular function is assessed visually as well as by measuring physiologic parameters such as end diastolic and systolic volumes, stroke volume, ejection fractions, etc., using a computer program.

Immediately following left ventriculography, left ventricular pressures are usually found to be significantly elevated. However, hearts in marked left ventricular failure with or without aneurysms may show little if any elevation of end diastolic pressure following left ventriculography. On the other hand, patients with normal cardiac functions may show a significant rise of end diastolic pressure following injection of contrast medium.

The left ventricular catheter is replaced by the left coronary artery catheter. If the proper sized catheter is selected, catheterization is accomplished. The catheter is connected to a transparent, polyvinyl tubing which allows observation of air bubbles. In addition, continuous pressure monitoring may be carried out; but in Amplatz's experience it is not necessary because it may give erroneous results, particularly if the catheter tip lies against the wall of the coronary artery. Pressure tracings may, therefore, be dampened without significant obstruction. Two important tests are carried out in order to assure a nonobstructing catheter:

1. A small test injection made under fluoroscopic control should show immediate clearing of contrast medium from the injected coronary artery. (If coronary artery occlusion should be present, this clearing may be delayed and should be readily recognized by the fluoroscopist).
2. There should be free back flow of flushing solution from the transparent connecting tubing when the syringe is disconnected. This free backflow is checked every fifteen to twenty seconds.

The electrocardiogram is continuously monitored. One should not, however, depend upon the electrocardiogram to recognize occlusion of the coronary artery by the catheter.

Six to ten cc of Renografin 60 or 76* are injected manually.

* Manufactured by Squibb.

It is of paramount importance to choose a contrast medium with an adequate concentration of sodium. Contrast media with low sodium content (Reno M 60 or 76* and Hypaque 60†) should not be used since they may induce ventricular fibrillation. Renografin 76 until now has been shown to be less toxic and to produce less cardiac arrythmias.[6,7]

Radiológraphic Technique

At least three injections are made in the left anterior oblique, right anterior oblique, and lateral positions. For cine recording a cradle can be used, but for radiographic imaging with a single plane film changer, a simple turning device may prove helpful. The patient is simply rotated by a motor driven Mylar belt and immobilized by a cloth harness.

The roentgenographic technique differs from that of Sones who does not obtain radiographic film recording of the injected coronary arteries. Whether filming or cine angiography is selected depends largely on the available facilities since both techniques have advantages. The obvious advantage of radiographic filming is its higher resolution and the possibility of studying a lesion in various projections at leisure. This is particularly important to the operating surgeon who will be taking the "road map" to the operating room.

Another advantage of film recording is exact measurement of atherosclerotic lesions. The coronary artery proximal and distal to an area of stenosis can be measured exactly, and the degree of narrowing can be expressed in percentages. By measuring the outside diameter of the catheter on the radiographic image, the magnification factor can be determined from a chart, thus absolute measurements in millimeters can be given as far as size of coronary arteries or areas of stenoses are concerned.

Although it is not known with certainty what percentage of coronary artery stenosis is hemodynamically significant, particularly under exercise, it is generally agreed that a degree of narrowing less than 50 per cent does not represent a good indication for surgical bypass.

* Manufactured by Squibb.
† Manufactured by Winthrop.

Cine recording, on the other hand, has the advantage of being more convenient and faster which is of particular importance to the patient's safety. The results can immediately be seen on the television monitor or recorded on magnetic tape. Hemodynamic events, as for instance narrowing by myocardial bridges, are usually better seen by cine coronary arteriography; but anatomic definition is still inferior to radiographic filming.

One of the main drawbacks of film recording is the cumbersome placement of the patient over the film changer. An additional problem is leaving the catheter inside the coronary ostium until the patient has been placed over the film changer which, however, has been shown to be innocuous.[8] Both problems have been overcome by the construction of a see-through changer which can be used similarly to a cine camera[9] (see Fig. 8).

Generally speaking, radiographic recording of coronary arteriograms on film is technically more difficult than cine recording. The major technical difficulties are unsharpness due to continuous motion of the heart, secondary radiation, and geometric unsharpness due to the use of high MA settings and large focal spot tubes. The following general guidelines will be helpful:

a) Exposure times should be short, ideally 1 msec to 3 msec, but in practical coronary arteriography 8 msec to 12 msec exposures will suffice.

b) A small focal spot tube, ideally of 0.3 mm dimension, will give the best results. At the present time, however, the heat capacity of fractional focal spot tubes limits their use to slender patients. A good compromise is, therefore, the use of a 0.6 mm focal spot tube.

c) Motion unsharpness should be minimized by placing the heart close to the film changer.

d) Secondary radiation is minimized by maximal coning, greatly facilitated by the use of a see-through changer. An 8:1 grid is desirable.

e) A combination of high speed screens and high speed film should be used.

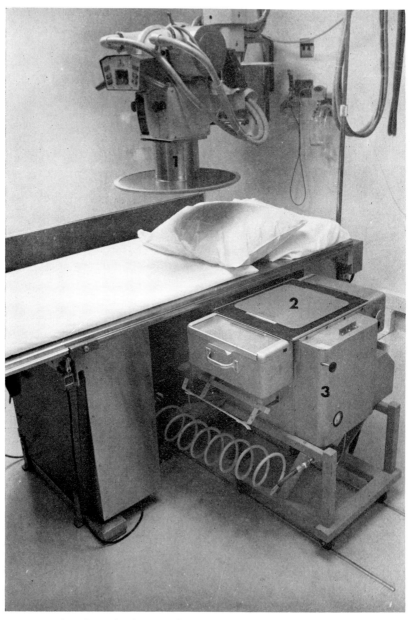

Figure 8. See-through changer developed by Amplatz. 1—Collimator with round shield to absorb scatter radiation. 2—See-through changer fitting under the floating table top, and over the image amplifier.[3]

f) The x-ray tube is placed in immediate contact with the patient, resulting in desirable magnification of approximately 1.5.[10] By doing so, the target film distance can be decreased to 28 to 32 inches, thus gaining penetration because of the inverse square law.

THE JUDKINS TECHNIQUE

Also inspired by Ricketts and Abrams, Judkins developed right and left coronary catheters which are now manufactured by Cordis Corp., Miami, Florida.

The left coronary catheter is shaped as seen in Figure 9. The body of the catheter is 8 French, has a 12 strand braid of stainless steel wire incorporated into its wall, and a 0.056 inch internal diameter. The material utilized is polyurethane. The rounded tips are 1.8 mm in diameter and have an 18 mm length with no side holes.

The catheter has a primary angle of about 90 degrees (see Fig. 9 (1)), a secondary angle of about 180 degrees (see Fig. 9 (2)), and the radius of the tertiary curve is about 10 cm in length (see Fig. 9 (3)). The standard size (#4) has a secondary portion which measures 4.2 cm, the #5 (used for dilated aortas) has a secondary portion which measures 5.2 cm, and the #6 (used for post-stenotic dilatation) has a secondary portion* measuring 6 cm. In addition, whereas the radius of the tertiary curve remains the same for all sizes, the primary curve angle (see Fig. 9 (1)) varies from 100 degrees to 90 degrees to 80 degrees for sizes 4, 5, and 6. The secondary curve angle varies from 160 degrees to 180 degrees to 200 degrees for the same corresponding sizes (see Fig. 9 (2)).

The catheter is introduced through the femoral artery over a Teflon coated guide wire. The catheter is maneuvered into the ascending aorta over the guide, at which time the guide is removed and the catheter assumes a "relaxed" position in the aortic arch. The patient is then turned into a 20 degree right posterior oblique projection and the catheter is slowly advanced

* The secondary portion is the portion between the primary and secondary curves (see Fig. 9 (2)).

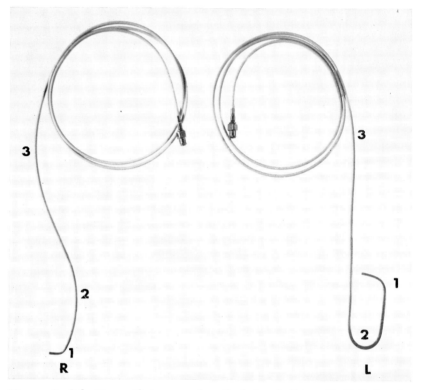

Figure 9. Selective catheters as described by Judkins. R—Catheter for the right coronary artery. L—Catheter for the left coronary artery. 1—Primary curve. 2—Secondary curve. 3—Tertiary curve.

until it drops into the coronary orifice. The spring afforded by the secondary bend holds the tip in the coronary orifice (see Fig. 10). Figure 11 demonstrates well why a catheter of varying lengths must be used when the ascending aorta is large or small.

The right coronary catheter (see Fig. 9) is manufactured in three sizes. Again, the secondary portion (see Fig. 9 (2)) measures either 4 cm, 5 cm, or 6 cm. The primary curve (see Fig. 9 (1)) remains 95 degrees for all sizes as does the secondary curve which measures 30 degrees (see Fig. 9 (2)). The catheter is advanced to a point about 2 cm to 3 cm above the left coronary orifice, then it is rotated slowly 180 degrees

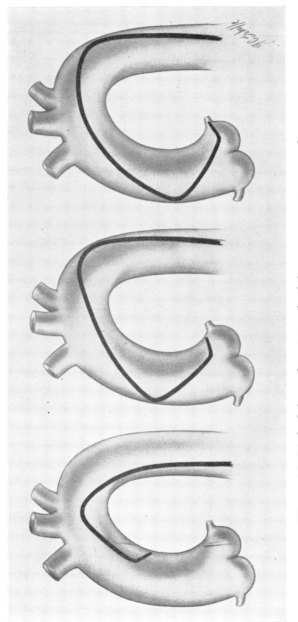

Figure 10. Method for catheterizing the left coronary artery according to Judkins.

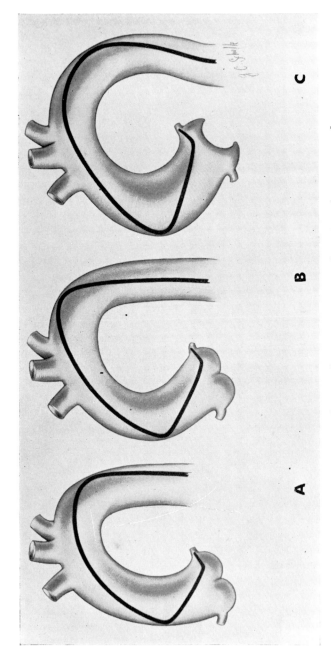

Figure 11. A, Normal ascending aorta, a number 4 catheter is used. B, Slightly tortuous ascending aorta, a number 5 catheter is used. C, Markedly tortuous aorta, a number 6 catheter is used.

until it drops into the right coronary orifice (see Fig. 12). The curve of the aortic arch causes the catheter to descend toward the right coronary ostium as it is rotated. If the catheter does not enter the right coronary artery on the first try, the level of rotation should be adjusted; up (if the catheter tip descends deep into the sinus of Valsalva), or down (if the tip rotates above the lip of the right coronary artery). Figure 13 demonstrates the need for different catheter shapes when the aorta widens.

Selective injections of 6 to 8 cc of Renografin 76 are delivered by hand and films of the left coronary artery are obtained in the left lateral, left anterior oblique, and right anterior oblique positions with the patient placed against a lateral film changer. The same amount of contrast is injected and identical projections are used for the right coronary artery. Both overframed motion picture films at 60 frames per second and rapid serial films at 4 per second for two seconds, and one per second for two seconds are obtained. Myocardial function is also evaluated by ventriculography. The Judkins'[11] "pig tail" catheter is used for the opacification of the left ventricle.

Judkins very emphatically stresses that cine angiography should be combined with direct serial radiography. He recommends obtaining the following equipment:[12]

1. A 3 phase 1,000 MA 12 pulse generator is to be used because it allows short exposure times while maintaining voltage in the 70 to 95 KV range. The focal spot should usually not exceed 1.2 mm.
2. The procedure is to be performed in a well-equipped cardiovascular laboratory where electrocardiographic as well as pressure recordings and defibrillating equipment are available.
3. The contrast medium utilized is Meglumine Diatrizoate 76% (Renografin 76) which in Judkins' laboratory has not produced a single case of arrhythmia in over 3,000 contrast injections (1970).

In order to obtain diagnostic films the radiologist should supervise the radiographic technique. One important factor is

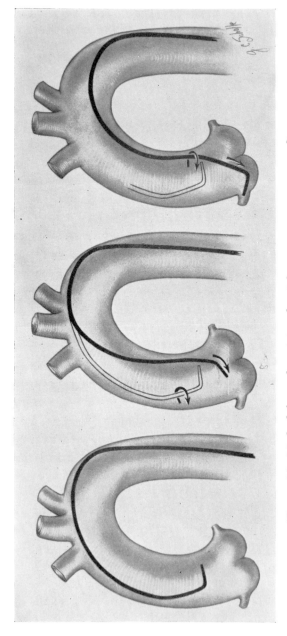

Figure 12. Method for catheterizing the right coronary artery according to Judkins.

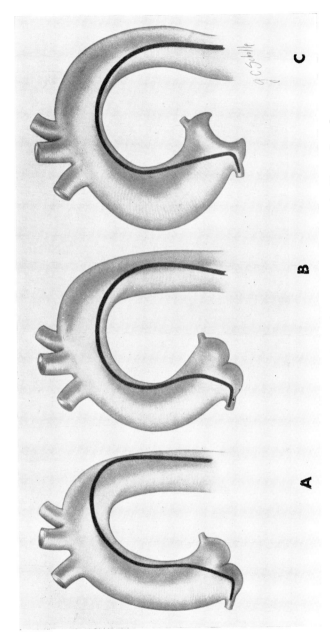

Figure 13. Catheterization of the right coronary ostium. A, Normal arch, a number 4 catheter is used. B, Slightly dilated arch, a number 5 catheter is used. C, Markedly widened aorta, a number 6 catheter is used. Drawings of figures 10 through 13 were provided by Dr. Melvin Judkins.

to have excellent screen film contact. If a stationary grid is used, as it is with most commercially available film changers, the grid line should be easily seen.

Biplane radiography, in adult patients, should be discouraged, because of the excessive scattering radiation.

Premedication of the Patients

The patients are premedicated with Seconal (100 mg), Phenergan (25 mg), and Atropine (0.6 mg), (all administered intramuscularly). The Atropine is supposed to reduce the vagal response to the procedure.

Others prefer to give 1 mg. of Atropine intravenously at the first sign of vagal response. This usually manifests itself by producing tiredness, sweating, yawning, and finally bradycardia and hypotension. The early manifestations of vagal effect must be immediately recognized and treated, otherwise it may result in an irreversible vaso-vagal response.

Judkins almost routinely uses nitroglycerine during the procedure. He feels, as Sones does, that it gives better visualization of the coronaries. Whereas Sones prescribes "Isordil"* routinely prior to the procedure, Judkins prefers nitroglycerine because of the short duration of its action (10 to 15 minutes).

At times one may select the wrong size catheter. If the catheter is too small, it will double up in the ascending aorta and if it is too large, the tip will tend to rest on the lip of the sinus of Valsalva. The *right* catheter is somewhat more difficult to introduce into the ostium of the coronary artery and the operator has to learn to judge when to rotate the catheter from left to right (see Fig. 12). Whereas the Amplatz catheter spontaneously tends to point anteriorly, the Judkins' right coronary catheter points towards the left. The tip of the catheter is small and has a "bullet nose" shape which should prevent it from damaging the coronary artery. Occasionally, the catheter will spring into a partially stenosed ostium and will occlude it. This is more likely to occur on the right side.

* IVES Laboratories, Inc.

The general rules described previously also apply here. Thus, one must immediately withdraw the catheter when the contrast fails to clear during a test injection or when damping of the pressure is noted. In those instances, the catheter must be manipulated until its position permits free flow of blood around it. Failure to apply this rule may result in dire complications. At times, however, it is impossible to catheterize the coronary ostium without occluding it, particularly when the ostium is stenotic. In such a situation, a rapid injection of contrast is immediately recorded on motion picture film and the catheter then quickly withdrawn. When this maneuver is utilized both the operator and the patient may suffer from angina!

Although the catheter manufacturer recommends disposal of the catheters after they have been used, it is common practice to reutilize them many times. Judkins feel that it is important to reshape such catheters with special wires* by immersing them in boiling water for at least two minutes. However, since polyurethane with incorporated wire mesh has such excellent memory, we have not felt the need for reshaping our catheters before reutilization. Silicone solutions can also be injected into the lumen of the catheter in order to facilitate introduction of the guide wire. Gas sterilization is necessary.

Lately polyethylene catheters with incorporated stainless steel bands have become available, shaped as described by Judkins.†

NEW YORK HOSPITAL TECHNIQUE

The "Amplatz" or "Judkins" catheters are used according to the individual cases. In some instances, one shape might be more suitable than the other and thus both techniques should be learned. In case of severe atherosclerosis of the iliac vessels, we also utilize Sones' technique by percutaneous transaxillary approach. Lately, we have given preference to catheters made

---

* Shaping wires available by Cath Aids, 4308 S.E. 35 Ave., Portland, Oregon 97202.

† Made by Cook, Inc., 925 S. Curry Pike, Bloomington, Ind. 47401.

of polyethylene with incorporated mesh* with the assumption
that they are less thrombogenic.

The patients are not premedicated and Valium is only administered when the patients are very anxious. This happens
rather rarely in our hospital.

Nitroglycerine is only given when the patient complains of
angina or if spasm is suspected. We believe that administration
of nitroglycerin in patients with coronary disease may produce
significant hypotension. This has already occurred in our laboratory. Furthermore, nitroglycerin should certainly not be
given before physiologic data has been obtained (LVED pres-
sures-cardiac output-myocardial function tests).

Currently, we administer routinely 1 mg of Atropine intramuscularly prior to starting the procedure. This presents a
twofold advantage: a) It reduces the bradycardia and the drop
of ventricular pressure during the injection of contrast material
and b) At least experimentally in dogs when Atropine is administered, the intracoronary injection of microemboli is better
tolerated.[13]

Catheterization of the coronary arteries is done with constant monitoring of pressures using a setup as shown in Figure
14. If the pressure drops while the catheter tip is in the coronary artery, the catheter is immediately pulled back.

The study is done in the following sequence:

1. A selective right coronary catheter is introduced into the
   left ventricle where baseline pressure recordings are obtained. The physiologic data should always be gathered
   prior to the injection of contrast medium. The patient
   is then placed into the left anterior oblique projection
   and the catheter is introduced into the right coronary
   artery.† With the patient in this position, a cine angiogram is performed injecting 6 cc to 8 cc of Renografin
   76 manually. He is then moved to the lateral film changer
   maintaining the same position. Using a horizontal x-ray

---

* Made by Cook, Inc., 9255 Curry Pike, Bloomington, Ind. 47401.
  † Catheterization of both coronary arteries is easiest with the patient in the
LAO position.

beam and the lateral changer, overhead radiographs are obtained. This results in films in the right anterior oblique projection.

2. The right coronary catheter is left in place and the patient is returned to the image amplifier. If the catheter has remained in the coronary ostium, the patient is turned into the right anterior oblique projection. A cine angiogram is then obtained in this new position. Without

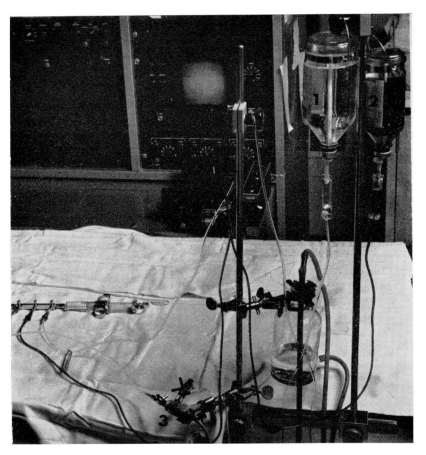

Figure 14. Set-up used at New York Hospital. 1. G/ 5% + Heparin (10,000 Units in 1 liter). 2. Contrast (Renografin 76). 3. Pressure transducer.

moving either the catheter or the patient, the table top is moved to the lateral film changer and overhead films are exposed using the horizontal beam. This results in the left anterior oblique view.

The catheter is then pulled back into the descending aorta and the films are developed in a 90 second X-omat* processor.

3. After viewing the right coronary arteriogram, the same process is repeated for the left coronary artery.

4. A pigtail ventricular catheter is introduced into the left ventricle. The patient is placed into the right anterior oblique projection and 40 cc to 50 cc of contrast are injected at a rate of 16 cc to 22 cc/sec. A cine angiogram is obtained at 60 frames/sec. Often left ventriculography in the left anterior oblique projection is also performed to view the septum and the lateral wall of the ventricle.

We are now considering the use of a 105 mm camera instead of a film changer. With the advent of better image amplifiers and cameras taking up to 6 exposures per second, it is conceivable that the radiographic detail will be acceptable (see Fig. 15) in which case we will spare a great deal of radiation and we will be able to obtain good films as easily as cine angiograms.

Prior to pulling the catheter back, a left ventricular pressure recording is obtained again.

The entire procedure is usually terminated within 45 to 60 minutes.

A coronary angiogram must not only give anatomic detail, but also it must provide physiologic data. Thus, with the advent of coronary artery surgery, it is important to obtain information regarding ventricular function. The ventriculogram alone is a poor indicator of myocardial function.

Left ventricular end diastolic pressures are often used as a

---

* Made by Kodak.

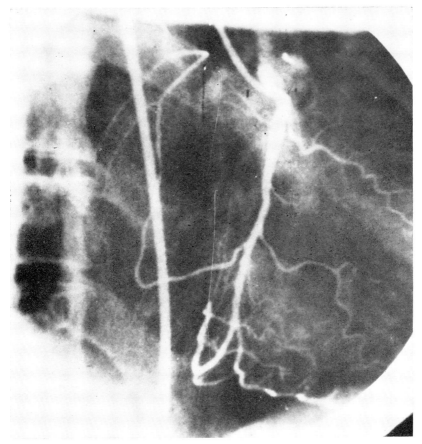

Figure 15. Right coronary arteriogram obtained with a 70 mm camera (This case has been lent to us by Robert Crawford of Siemens, Inc.).

reliable myocardial function test; however, these pressures may be elevated due to other reasons than myocardial dysfunction: hypovolemia, valvular disease, circulatory shunts, and pericardial effusion.[14] At New York Hospital some surgeons rely heavily on this measurement for assessing ventricular function. Gensini *et al.*[15] and more recently Levin *et al.*[16] have shown that the injection of contrast into the coronary arteries raises the end diastolic pressure considerably, particularly if myocardial function is compromised (see Fig. 16). Thus we recommend that pressure measurements in the heart and other physiologic tests be performed prior to angiography. Some believe that ventriculography should be carried out prior to coronary angiography because the contrast might adversely influence ventricular function and impair the quality of contraction. However, we prefer to perform coronary angiography first.

OTHER VARIOUS METHODS

Other percutaneous methods have been described and will only be cited below for general interest. The reader is referred

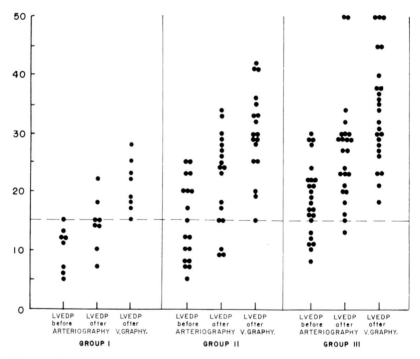

Figure 16. Diagram demonstrating the effect of contrast medium upon the myocardium during coronary angiography and left ventriculography. Group I—Normal patients. Group II—Patients with diseased coronary arteries but normal ventriculograms. Group III—Patients with diseased coronary arteries and abnormal ventriculograms. Note the elevation of pressure following the injection of contrast material. The elevation is more marked in patients in Groups II and III.

to the original articles since the authors do not have personal experience with those techniques.

Weidner modified Sones' technique and recommended the transaxillary approach.[17] Polyethylene catheters were used in conjunction with a Muller USCI guide system.*

Originally, Viamonte[18] developed a guide system to be used with a Ducor catheter.

Bourassa[19] described lately a new set of coronary catheters made of polyethylene.*

Many angiographers prefer to use preshaped catheters and since the Ducor catheter has become available, coronary angiography has become a very easy procedure. Either the Amplatz, the Judkins, the Bourassa, or Sones catheters will give satisfactory results provided the operator has some experience with catheterization procedures.

REFERENCES

1. Ricketts, H.J., and Abrams, H.L.: Percutaneous selective coronary cine arteriography, *J.A.M.A.*, *181*:620–24, 1962.
2. Amplatz, K., Formanek, G., Stranger, P., and Wilson, W.: Mechanics of selective coronary artery catheterization via femoral approach. *Radiology*, *89*:1040–47, 1967.
3. Wilson, W.J., Lee, G.B., and Amplatz, K.: Biplane selective coronary arteriography via percutaneous transfemoral approach. *Am. J. Roentgen.*, *100*:332–340, 1967.
4. Judkins, M.P.: Selective coronary arteriography I. A percutaneous transfemoral technic. *Radiology*, *89*:815–24, 1967.
5. Amplatz, K.: Technics of coronary arteriography. *Circulation*, *27*:101–106, 1963.
6. Gensini, G., DiGiorgi, S.: Myocardial toxicity of contrast agents used in angiography. *Radiology*, *82/1*:24–34, 1964.
7. Paulin, S. and Adams, F.D.: Increased ventricular fibrillation during coronary arteriography with a new contrast medium preparation. *Radiology*, *101*:45–50, 1971.
8. Baltaxe, H.A., Formanek, G., Loken, M., Amplatz, K.: Clinical limitations to use of Xenon for measurement of myocardial blood flow. *Invest. Radiol.*, *4/5*:317–322, 1969.
9. Amplatz, K.: New rapid roll-film changer. *Radiology*, *90/1*:130–34, 1968.

* Manufactured by United States Catheter and Instrument Corp.

10. Randall, A.P., and Amplatz, K.: Magnification coronary arteriography. *Radiology, 101*:51–56, 1971.

11. Boijsen, E., Judkins, M.P.: A hook tail "closed end" catheter for percutaneous selective cardioangiography. *Radiology, 87*:872–877, 1966.

12. Judkins, M.P.: Percutaneous transfemoral selective coronary arteriography. *Radiol. Clin. N. Am., VI/3*, Dec. 1968.

13. Guzman, S.V., Swenson, E., Mitchell, R.: Mechanism of cardiogenic shock. *Circ. Res., 10*:746, 1962.

14. Braunwald, E. and Ross, J.: The ventricular end diastolic pressure. Appraisal of its value in recognition of ventricular failure in man. *Am. J. Med., 34*:147–150, 1963.

15. Gensini, G.G., Dubiel, J., Huntington, P.P., Kelly, A.E.: Left ventricular end-diastolic pressure before and after coronary arteriography. *Am. J. Cardiol., 27*:453–459, 1971.

16. Levin, D.C. and Baltaxe, H.A.: The effects of selective coronary arteriography upon left ventricular function as manifested by left ventricular end diastolic pressure. Exhibited at the 72nd Annual Meeting of American Roentgen Ray Society 1971. *N.Y.S.J. of Med. 72*: 2619, 1972.

17. Weidner, W., Mac Alpin, R., Hanafee, W., *et al.*: Percutaneous transaxillary selective coronary angiography. *Radiology, 85*:652–657, 1965.

18. Viamonte, M., Jr., Gosselin, A.J., Sommer, L.S.: Coronary arteriography: Some observations on technique and interpretation. *Am. J. Roentgen., 92*:872–876, 1964.

19. Bourassa, M.G., Lespérance, J., and Campeau, L.: Selective coronary arteriography by the percutaneous femoral artery approach. *Am. J. Roentgen., 107*:377, 1969.

CHAPTER IV

ANATOMY OF THE NORMAL CORONARY ARTERY TREE—ANGIOGRAPHIC ANATOMY

The purpose of this chapter is to describe the anatomy of the normal coronary artery tree, and to explain its arteriographic appearance as it is seen in the various projections commonly used during coronary angiography.

It is of paramount importance for the angiographer to be entirely familiar with normal coronary artery patterns and their variations. There is a wide range of anatomical and positional variations making interpretations of coronary arteriograms sometimes very difficult.

The coronary arteries arise from the sinuses of Valsalva through ostia which generally are located in the center of the sinus (see Fig. 17). It is, however, not uncommon to see ostia displaced towards the adjacent commissures. The shape of the coronary ostium is usually oval or round and measures from 0.7 to 1.5 cm in diameter. The angle between the coronary arteries and the aortic wall as a rule is 90 degrees, but in older hearts, this angle may be markedly diminished producing a very sharp turn. There may be multiple orifices for the various branches of each artery rendering selective catheterization difficult (see Chap. V). The aortic sinus of Valsalva is that portion of the aorta which is found between the sino-tubular ridge and the aortic valve leaflets. This sinotubular ridge is an important landmark for selective coronary arteriography. It can be easily identified with a catheter. If one introduces a catheter with a slight distal curve into the ascending aorta to the level of the aortic valve leaflets and pulls it back gently, eventually the catheter will bounce off the sino-tubular ridge.

Contrary to popular belief, the aortic sinuses are not of exactly the same size since the posterior or noncoronary sinus is usually slightly larger than the left sinus (see Fig. 17). Unfortunately, the nomenclature of the sinuses is misleading since in the anteroposterior position, the right coronary sinus lies in the right anterolateral position, the left sinus lies in the left posterolateral position, and the noncoronary sinus lies in the right posterolateral position (see Fig. 17). Consequently, if catheteri-

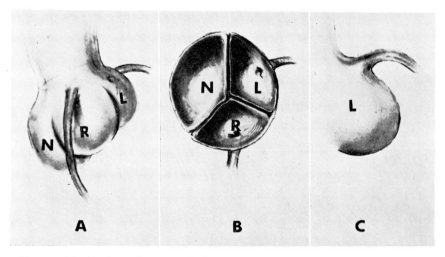

Figure 17. A, Frontal view of the cast of an ascending aorta demonstrating well the origin of each coronary artery. B, Horizontal view of the same cast. Note that the right (R) coronary artery arises anteriorly whereas the left coronary artery (L) arises to the left and posteriorly. Also see that the noncoronary cusp (N) is larger than the others. C, Cast positioned to simulate a patient's aorta in the left anterior oblique projection. The proximal portion of the left coronary artery is well seen in this fashion. This is also the best position for intubating either coronary artery.

zation of the right coronary artery is done in the anteroposterior projection, it is accomplished by pointing the catheter almost directly towards the operator in the sagittal plane rather than towards the right.

THE LEFT CORONARY ARTERIAL TREE

The Main Left Coronary Artery

The left main coronary artery is a short trunk arising from the left aortic sinus running from its ostium through the aortic wall towards the left and anteriorly in the anterior atrioventricular sulcus. It is covered anteriorly by the auricle of the left atrium. The main trunk varies considerably in size ranging from a few millimeters to 4 cm. As a rule, the left main coronary artery bifurcates into the left anterior descending and circumflex coronary arteries. On occasion, it may trifurcate, giving rise to left anterior descending, circumflex and diagonal arteries.

Angiographic Anatomy

The left main coronary artery is often comparatively free of atherosclerosis and consequently obstruction of this vessel by the selective catheter is uncommon. On the anteroposterior and lateral projections (see Figs. 18 and 19), the left main coronary artery has an almost horizontal course, differing from the right coronary artery which swings slightly upwards. It is important to realize that in the AP view and in the right anterior oblique projection the left main coronary artery appears foreshortened and its orifice is usually not visualized. In the left anterior oblique projection, the orifice of the left main coronary artery is seen in profile, allowing visualization of the most proximal portion of that artery (see Fig. 20). Thus cases of main left coronary artery stenosis will be missed if the LAO projection is overlooked. On the other hand, the right anterior oblique projection often demonstrates the more distal segment of the left coronary artery just prior to its bifurcation (see Fig. 21). Figures 22 and 23 also demonstrate the same points on an actual angiogram.

The Left Circumflex Coronary Artery

This vessel is a branch of the left main coronary artery. It may vary considerably in size depending upon whether the posterior descending artery is a branch of the right (right pre-

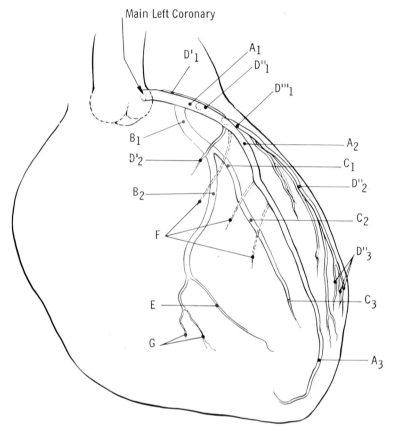

Left Coronary Artery

A - Ant. Descending Coronary A.   E - Diaphragmatic Branches
B - Circumflex Coronary Artery   (Postero Lateral Branches)
C - Obtuse Marginal Artery   F - Septal Branches
D - Diagonal Arteries   G - Atrio.Ventricular Branch
                                  of Circumflex Artery

Figure 18. Diagram of a left coronary arteriogram seen in the anteroposterior projection. Refer to the code to identify vessels. Note that each point on this drawing corresponds to the same point on Figure 19.

Left Coronary Artery

A - Ant. Descending Coronary A.   E - Diaphragmatic Branches
B - Circumflex Coronary Artery   (Postero Lateral Branches)
C - Obtuse Marginal Artery   F - Septal Branches
D - Diagonal Arteries   G - Atrio.Ventricular Branch
                                         of Circumflex Artery

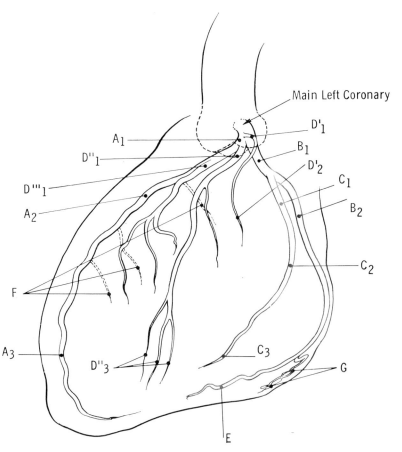

Figure 19. Diagram of a selective left coronary arteriogram seen in the lateral position (same patient as in Figure 18).

Left Coronary Artery

A - Ant. Descending Coronary A.	E - Diaphragmatic Branches
B - Circumflex Coronary Artery	(Postero Lateral Branches)
C - Obtuse Marginal Artery	F - Septal Branches
D - Diagonal Arteries	G - Atrio.Ventricular Branch
	of Circumflex Artery

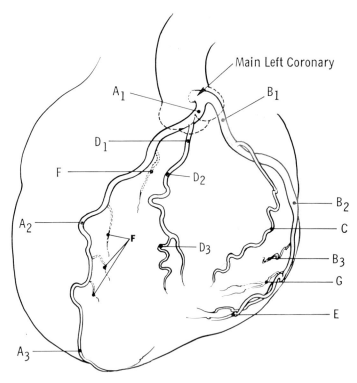

Figure 20. Diagram of a left coronary arteriogram in the left anterior oblique projection. Same patient as in Figure 21.

Left Coronary Artery

A - Ant. Descending Coronary A.
B - Circumflex Coronary Artery
C - Obtuse Marginal Artery
D - Diagonal Arteries

E - Diaphragmatic Branches
   (Postero Lateral Branches)
F - Septal Branches
G - Atrio.Ventricular Branch
   of Circumflex Artery

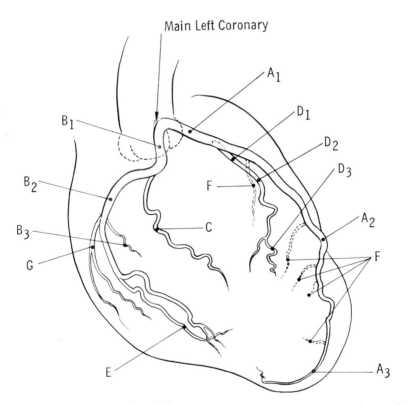

Figure 21. Diagram of a left coronary arteriogram seen in the right anterior oblique projection. Refer to the code to identify the vessels. Note that this is the same patient as in Figure 20.

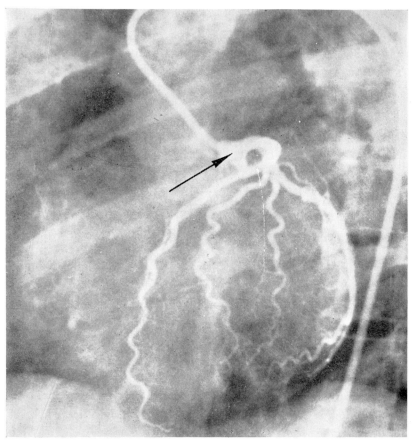

Figure 22. Left anterior projection of a selective left coronary angiogram. Note how well the orifice of the left coronary artery is seen (see arrow).

ponderant pattern—see Figs. 24 and 25) or circumflex (left preponderant pattern—see Figs. 26 and 27). In some individuals with strongly predominant right coronary arteries, the circumflex is very small or even absent. This should not be mistaken for atherosclerotic disease. The circumflex coronary artery measures generally 2 mm to 4 mm in external diameter. It courses forward under cover of the left auricular appendage and then curves to the left in the AV sulcus in front of the mitral valve. Running parallel to it and superficial or anterior to it is the great cardiac vein as it unites with the large atrial vein to form the origin of the coronary sinus.

Important branches arise from the circumflex coronary artery. The sinus node artery in approximately 50 per cent of cases is a

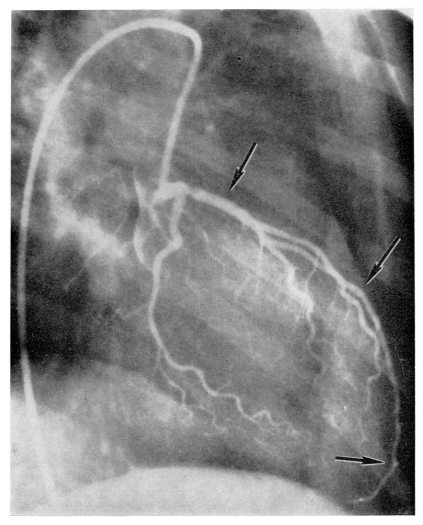

Figure 23. Right anterior oblique projection. The entire left anterior descending coronary artery is seen in profile and its course is marked by arrows. Note that the two angiograms in Figure 22 and 23 do not belong to the same patient as those described in the drawings.

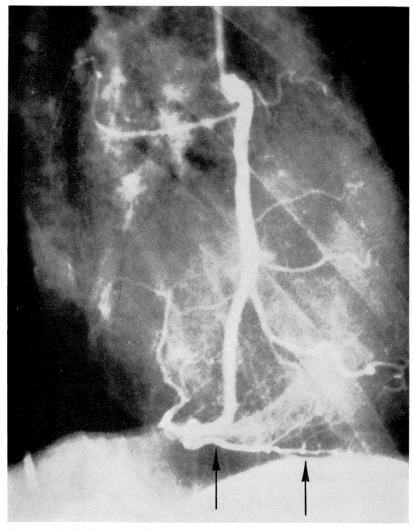

Figure 24. Right preponderant pattern. Right anterior oblique projection of a selective right coronary arteriogram. The posterior descending coronary artery arises from the right (see arrows). Figures 24 and 25 belong to the same patient. Diagramatic representation of the same arteriogram is seen in Figures 46 and 47.

branch of the circumflex coronary artery (see Figs. 28 and 54). It courses along the body of the anterior portion of the left atrium beneath the atrial appendage and reaches the anterior margin of the interatrial septum where it penetrates the septum. It then circles the base of the superior vena cava and vascularizes the sinus node.

Kugel's artery may also arise from the proximal portion of the circumflex coronary artery.[1] This vessel becomes an important collateral pathway when either right or left coronary arteries are occluded and supply of blood to the posterior left

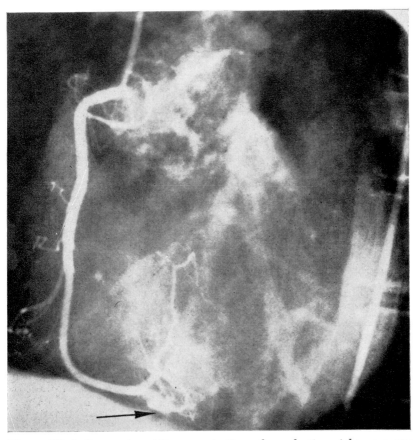

Figure 25. Left anterior oblique projection of a selective right coronary arteriogram. The posterior descending artery is seen foreshortened.

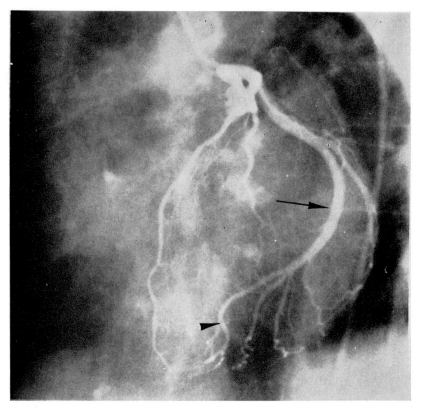

Figure 26. Left preponderant pattern. Left anterior oblique projection of a selective left coronary arteriogram. Note the large circumflex coronary artery (black arrow) giving rise to the posterior descending coronary artery (arrowhead).

ventricle comes from the ipsilateral side. Kugel's artery is a vessel which runs in the interatrial septum and arises either from the proximal right or the circumflex coronary artery (sometimes it may arise from the main left coronary artery) and connects those vessels to the AV node artery (see example of a Kugel's artery in Chapter VIII).

In some instances one of the major branches arising from the circumflex coronary artery is the left atrial circumflex artery (see Fig. 29). In cases of a dominant right coronary artery the atrial circumflex may be the only major branch arising from the

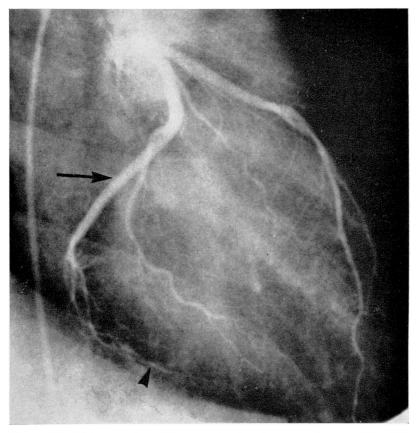

Figure 27. Right anterior oblique projection (same patient as Fig. 26). See the posterior descending coronary artery marked by black arrowhead. Black arrow points to the circumflex.

circumflex coronary artery. It supplies the lower portion of the left atrium and much of the left posterior atrial wall. It may also occasionally give rise to the sinus node artery.

Marginal branches are important branches arising from the left circumflex. They course towards the margo-obtusus and finally curve towards the apex of the heart. The largest of these branches, usually called the left marginal branch or the obtuse marginal branch, courses circumferentially around the lateral wall of the left ventricle. Distally on the diaphragmatic sur-

face, the circumflex coronary artery may divide into two or
three posterolateral muscular branches which perfuse the left
ventricle (see Figs. 18 through 21).

Angiographic Anatomy

The circumflex coronary artery is best seen on a lateral or
LAO projection. It is sometimes difficult to distinguish the cir-

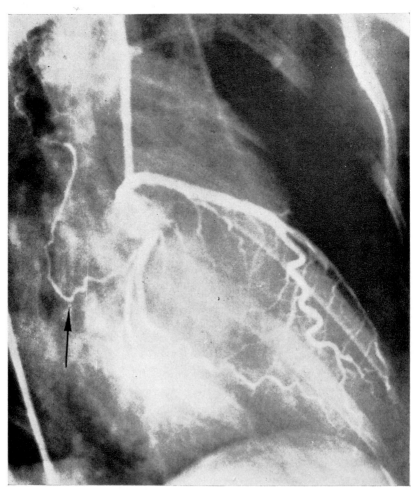

Figure 28. The sinus node artery (indicated by black arrow) arises
from the circumflex coronary artery.

cumflex artery from its marginal branch. The AP and RAO projections, however, may be helpful in distinguishing between the two. On the LAO projection (see Fig. 20), the circumflex artery proper courses to the left from the left coronary bifurcation and then it turns downward and slightly medially, following the atrioventricular groove. This helps distinguish it from the marginal branch which remains laterally positioned on this projection (see Figs. 20, 30, and 31). On the lateral film, however, the circumflex artery hugs the back of the heart (see Figs.

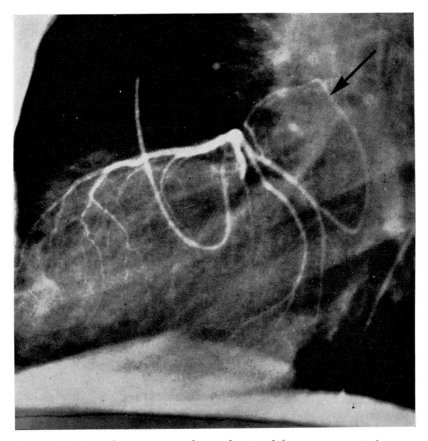

Figure 29. Lateral projection of a selective left coronary arteriogram. Note the large left atrial circumflex artery marked by the black arrow. This patient has mitral stenosis and therefore a large left atrium.

32 and 33), and is always posterior to the marginal branch. Also, the marginal branch, which runs over the lateral wall of the ventricle, is seen to be foreshortened during ventricular systole and demonstrates tortuosity. By contrast, the circumflex proper, which remains in the atrioventricular groove, does not fold like the bellows of an accordion during systole as does the marginal branch. The marginal branch is also easily identified on the RAO projection.

The sinus node artery and the left atrial circumflex artery,

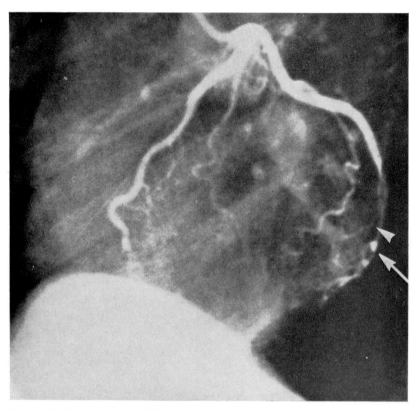

Figure 30. Left anterior oblique projection of a selective coronary arteriogram (same patient and same projection as Fig. 20). Note that the distal circumflex coronary artery is small (see white arrowhead) whereas the marginal branch (white arrow) is large and projects behind that vessel. Figures 30 and 31 are from the same patient.

when present, are best seen on the RAO or lateral projections where these vessels can be examined in their entirety (see Figs. 28 and 29). The posterior descending coronary artery when arising from the circumflex (dominant left) is best demonstrated on the RAO projection because it is not foreshortened as it may be on the LAO projection.

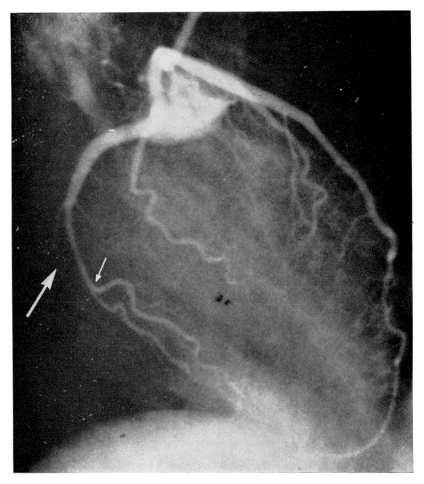

Figure 31. Right anterior oblique projection (same patient and projection as Fig. 21). The distal circumflex coronary artery is marked by the white arrow. The short white arrow points to the marginal branch.

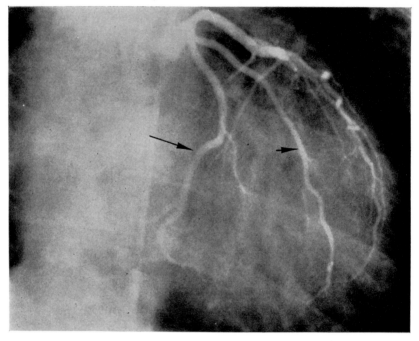

Figure 32. Antero-posterior view of a selective left coronary arteriogram. Dominant left pattern. Note the large circumflex coronary artery indicated by the black arrow. Short arrow points to the marginal branch.

The circumflex coronary artery may be extremely small or even appear absent when the posterior descending and left posterolateral arteries are completely supplied by the right coronary artery. In cases of balanced flow,[2,3] where the posterior descending and left posterolateral arteries originate partly from the circumflex and partly from the right coronary artery, the distal circumflex is of course of fairly large caliber.

Left Anterior Descending Coronary Artery

The left anterior descending is usually a direct continuation of the left main coronary artery. It runs in the anterior interventricular sulcus and thus varies in position depending on the presence of right or left ventricular hypertrophy (see Figs. 34

and 35). At times it may leave the interventricular groove and cross over the ventricle.[1] In some instances, there may be more than one anterior descending coronary artery. As it extends towards the apex of the heart it most commonly curves around it and enters the posterior interventricular sulcus to meet the posterior descending coronary artery (see Fig. 36).

The first branch of the left anterior descending coronary artery is the left conus artery which anastromoses with the right

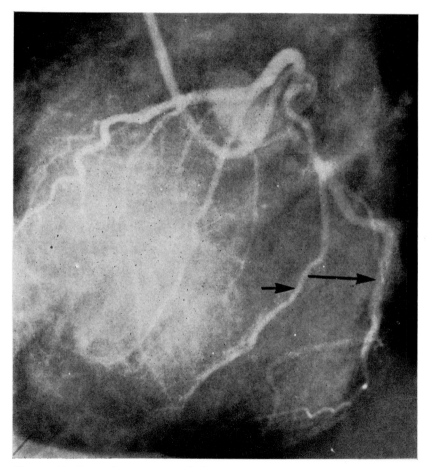

Figure 33. Lateral projection of the same arteriogram as in Figure 32. Note that the circumflex artery (long arrow) projects posterior to the marginal branch (short arrow).

conus artery, a branch of the right coronary artery. This represents an important anastomotic circle first described by Vieussens (Fig. 37).

The most important branches of the left anterior descending coronary artery are branches to the ventricular septum, the so-called anterior septal branches. These anterior septal branches anastomose with the posterior septal branches arising from the posterior descending artery. They are usually 4 to 6 arteries ex-

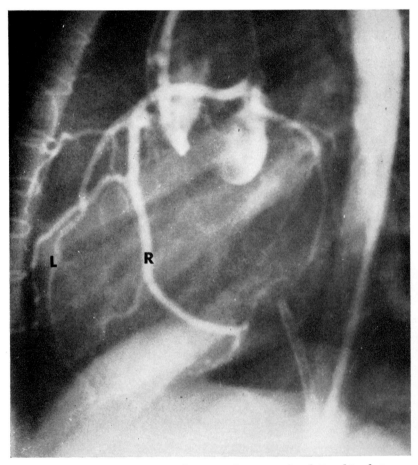

Figure 34. Lateral aortogram showing the normal relationship between the right coronary artery (R) and the left anterior descending coronary artery (L).

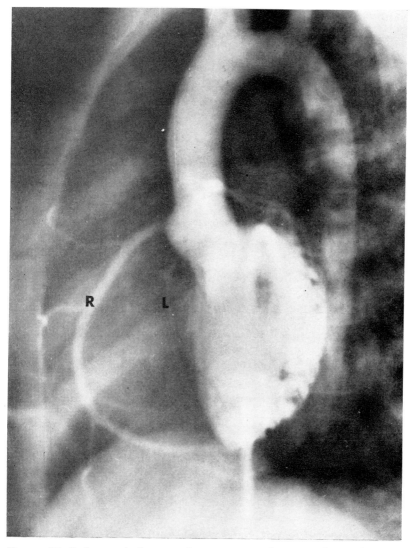

Figure 35. Left ventriculogram of a patient with an atrial septal defect. Note that the left anterior descending coronary artery (L) is posterior to the right coronary artery (R). This is due to right ventricular enlargement.

tending from the anterior descending artery straight into the anterior portion of the ventricular septum.

As it passes along its course, the anterior descending coronary artery also gives off muscular branches to both the left and right ventricles. These vessels are usually called diagonal branches and supply blood to the anterior surface of the infundibular part of the right ventricle as well as to the anterior surface of the left ventricle. These branches have a variable course and must not be mistaken for the anterior descending coronary artery itself.

Angiographic Anatomy

The anterior descending coronary artery is best seen in the RAO and lateral projections. It can be identified by the presence of the septal branches which tend to arise nearly perpen-

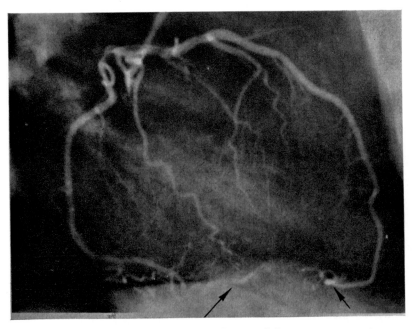

Figure 36. Lateral projection of a selective left coronary arteriogram. Dominant left pattern. Note that the left anterior descending coronary artery (short arrow) meets the posterior descending coronary artery (black arrow) in the posterior interventricular groove.

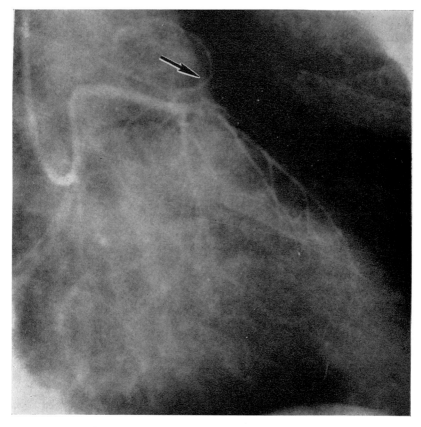

Figure 37. Right anterior oblique projection of a left coronary arteriogram. Note a large left conus branch shown with a black arrow.

dicularly from that vessel. In the lateral projection the left anterior descending coronary artery lies anterior to the right coronary artery (see Fig. 34). In cases of right ventricular enlargement, the left anterior descending coronary artery is pushed backward and its relationship to right coronary is reversed (see Fig. 35). In the LAO projection, the anterior descending coronary artery runs from top to bottom and from the patient's left to right in the middle of the cardiac shadow where the septum is seen on end. Diagonal branches may be mistaken for the anterior descending coronary artery, especially when they run close to the interventricular groove. The first septal branch often forms an acute angle with the anterior descending artery rather than a right angle. It may be very large when the anterior descending coronary artery is occluded, and it virtually always projects in the same area as the anterior descending artery in the LAO projection. Since this vessel runs within the septum and curves gently downward, it could be mistaken for the left anterior descending in the LAO projection. However, the difference will be apparent on the RAO projection (Figs. 38 and 39).

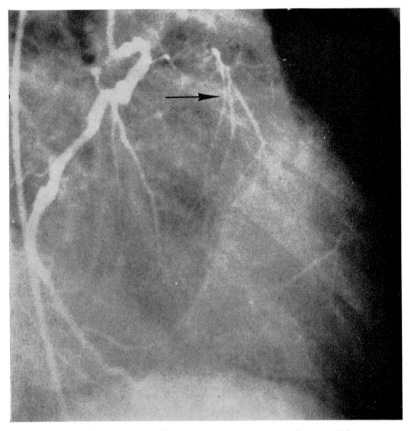

Figure 38. Right anterior oblique projection of a selective left coronary arteriogram. Note complete obstruction of the left anterior descending coronary artery. The septal branches, however, are visualized (black arrow). Figures 38 and 39 represent the same patient.

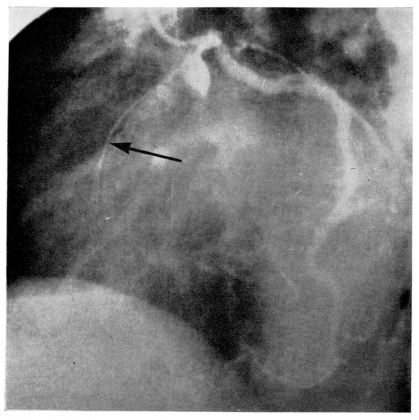

Figure 39. Left anterior oblique projection. The vessel running in the area where one would expect the left anterior descending artery to be is a septal branch (black arrow).

The Right Main Coronary Artery

After originating from the aorta this artery runs towards the right anteriorly behind the base of the pulmonary artery and under the right auricular appendage. It lies superior to the fibrous trigone, as well as the septal and anterior cusps of the tricuspid valve. The right coronary artery runs in the anterior atrioventricular groove until it reaches the acute margin of the heart where it turns posteriorly and caudally. It then continues its course in the atrioventricular groove to the diaphragmatic

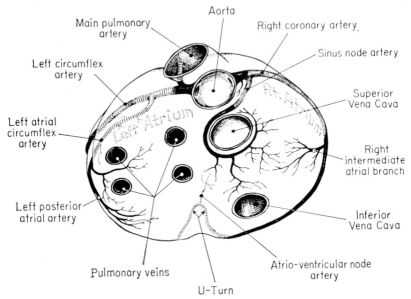

Figure 40. Diagramatic representation of the crown around the heart formed by the circumflex coronary artery and the right coronary artery.

surface of the heart. The right coronary artery and the circumflex coronary artery form a crown around the heart by encircling it totally (see Fig. 40).

In more than 50 per cent of the cases the first important branch of the right coronary artery is the right conal branch. In the other cases the right conal branch has its own separate origin from the right sinus of Valsalva.[4] The separate orifice of the conal branch, however, usually is in close proximity to the orifice of the right main coronary artery (see Fig. 41). The right conal branch anastomoses with the smaller left conal branch. This artery may be rather large, particularly in patients with congenital heart disease involving right ventricular hypertrophy, as for example in tetralogy of Fallot.

The next major branch arising from the right coronary artery is the sinus node artery which runs posteriorly and medially to the interatrial septum and then towards the superior vena cava (see Figs. 40 and 54). In its downward course, this vessel also supplies branches to the right atrium. Those atrial branches be-

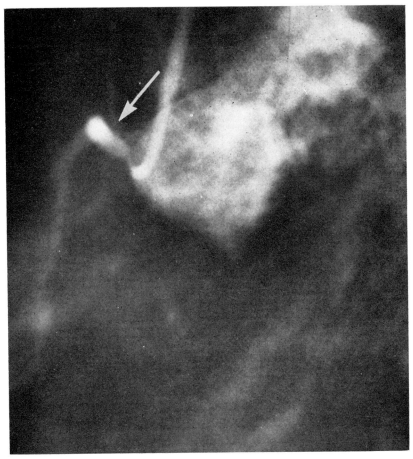

Figure 41. Cine frame of an injection into the right sinus of Valsalva. Left anterior oblique projection. Note the separate orifice of the conus branch (see arrow).

come a very important collateral pathway when the main right coronary artery is occluded (see Chap. VIII).

The right ventricular branches supply the free wall of the right ventricle. One of the most common and largest is a ventricular branch of the acute margin of the heart, also called the acute marginal branch. It supplies both the ventral and dorsal surfaces of the right ventricle. In addition to this main marginal branch, there are other small ventricular branches of lesser importance. After the right coronary artery reaches the acute margin of the heart, it continues along the right atrioventricular sulcus, winding posteriorly and medially towards the crux. At that point, it often forms an inverted U-shape and gives rise to the posterior descending artery.

In 90 per cent of cases, the posterior descending artery, which runs in the posterior interventricular sulcus, is a branch of the distal right coronary artery. This is the so-called "right preponderance." In only 10 per cent of cases, the posterior descending artery arises from the left circumflex artery and these are referred to as the left preponderant pattern. In patients with right preponderance, diaphragmatic myocardial infarctions are due to lesions of the right coronary artery.

The use of the term "right preponderance" is somewhat confusing and should not be taken to imply that most of the myocardium is being supplied by the right coronary artery. In all except the rare individuals with certain coronary artery anomalies, most of the left ventricular myocardium is supplied by branches of the left coronary artery. Preponderance only indicates which vessel supplies the posterior diaphragmatic surface of the left ventricle and the inferior portion of the interventricular septum.

The anatomy of the posterior descending artery is quite variable. Sometimes there are a number of diaphragmatic branches of the right coronary artery which terminate along the posterior interventricular sulcus.

The posterior descending artery supplies branches to the lower portion of the interventricular septum. These septal arteries extend in a cephalad direction towards the septal branches of the anterior descending artery. One of the most important septal branches is the artery to the AV node, which usually arises from the right coronary artery at the crux of the heart and passes cephalad to the node itself. Occasionally, the posterior septal branches do not arise from the posterior descending coronary artery, but from a large marginal branch[1] (see Figs. 42 and 43). To recognize this important anatomic varia-

tion becomes particularly critical when bypass surgery is contemplated.

In addition to the posterior descending coronary artery, the
distal right coronary gives off muscular branches which have
received various names. These branches supply blood to the
diaphragmatic wall of the right and left ventricles and usually
parallel the posterior descending coronary artery. They have
been called either right and left posterolateral branches or posterior right and posterior left ventricular branches. Their number and course varies and their size depends upon right or left
preponderance. Note that in the so-called balanced circulation,
the posterolateral branches arise from the circumflex coronary
artery.

Angiographic Anatomy

(See Figs. 44 through 47)

As already mentioned, the right coronary ostium points somewhat anteriorly and thus if the patient is catheterized in the
AP projection, the catheter must point directly at the operator.
This maneuver may be difficult and more time consuming than
if the patient is in the left anterior oblique position where the
ostium and the artery point directly to the right (left of the
operator). The two most common projections utilized are the
left anterior and right anterior oblique projections. The AP projection is less useful because of the overlying spine (see Fig.
48). The direct lateral projection is somewhat inferior to the
right anterior oblique projection as it foreshortens the collateral
pathways to the left anterior descending coronary artery when
those are present, and does not optimally demonstrate the posterior descending coronary artery.

In the left anterior oblique projection, the right coronary artery hugs the right border of the heart (see Fig. 49). In this
projection, the conus branch comes forward towards the pulmonary artery, whereas the sinus node branch bends medially
and posteriorly towards the superior vena cava. The muscular

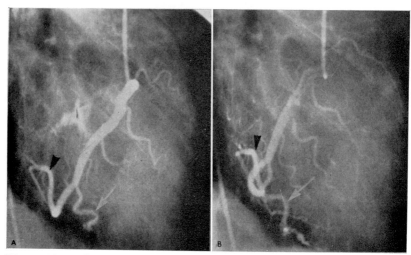

Figure 42. Right anterior oblique projection of a selective right coronary arteriogram. A, Early arterial phase. B, Late arterial phase. Note the large marginal branch indicated by the white arrow giving rise to posterior septal branches (seen in B). The arrowhead points to the distal right coronary artery.

branches and particularly the marginal branch usually remain to the right of the main coronary artery, also hugging the lateral portion of the cardiac shadow. In this projection, the marginal branch might be difficult to differentiate from the main right coronary artery as both appear to have a parallel course. Their identification becomes easy on the RAO projection (see Figs. 50 and 51). In the LAO and lateral projections, the crux is easily identified by the presence of the inverted "U." This U may not always be present. At the apex of the inverted U, one can see an opacified AV node artery. Occasionally, two AV node arteries are present (see Fig. 52). The fact that this vessel is not opacified does not mean that it is occluded. The posterior descending coronary artery is seen on end and is much foreshortened in these projections. It usually goes slightly downward and to the left as it courses in the interventricular groove. The better projection for good visualization of the posterior descending coronary artery is the RAO projection. Although the posterolateral branches are usually roughly parallel to the posterior descending coronary artery, they may not be quite as foreshortened in the LAO projection and one might see them very well at this time. This is because they do not remain within the septum and travel slightly towards the left (see Fig. 53).

In the right anterior oblique projection, the conus branch is usually well seen and easy to identify as it passes anteriorly over the pulmonary outflow tract. The sinus node artery if present is a major branch going posteriorly (see Fig. 54). The marginal

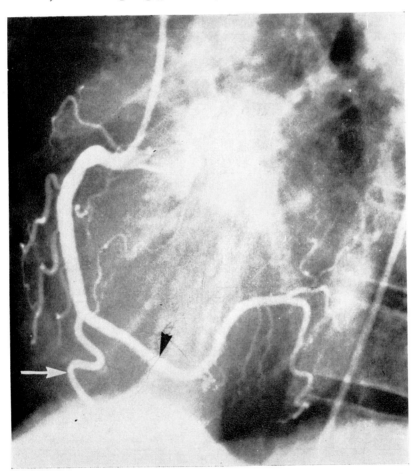

Figure 43. Left anterior oblique projection of the same patient as in Figure 42. Here also the arrow points to the marginal branch and the arrowhead to the distal right coronary artery.

Right Coronary Artery

A - Right Coronary Artery   F - Post. Descending Artery
B - SA Node Artery   G - AV Node Artery
C - Conus Artery   H - Septal Branches
D - Acute Marginal Artery   I - Postero Lateral Branches
E - Atrial Branch   K - Muscular Branches

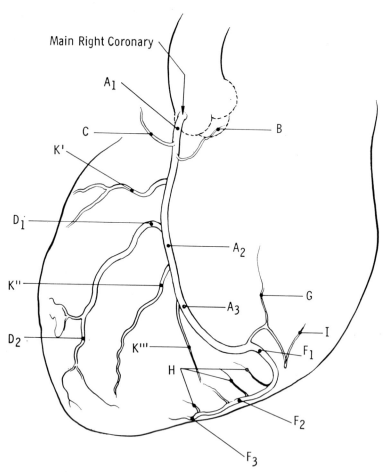

Figure 44. Diagramatic representation of a right coronary angiogram in the lateral projection.

Right Coronary Artery

A - Right Coronary Artery
B - SA Node Artery
C - Conus Artery
D - Acute Marginal Artery
E - Atrial Branch

F - Post. Descending Artery
G - AV Node Artery
H - Septal Branches
I - Postero Lateral Branches
K - Muscular Branches

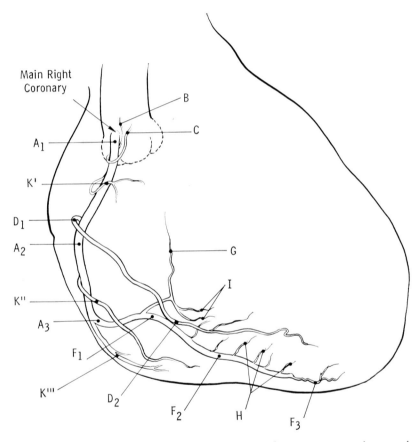

Figure 45. Diagramatic representation of a right coronary angiogram in the antero-posterior projection (same patient as Fig. 44).

Right Coronary Artery

A - Right Coronary Artery   F - Post. Descending Artery
B - SA Node Artery   G - AV Node Artery
C - Conus Artery   H - Septal Branches
D - Acute Marginal Artery   I - Postero Lateral Branches
E - Atrial Branch   K - Muscular Branches

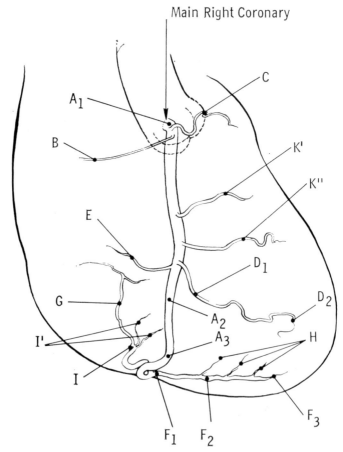

Figure 46. Diagramatic representation of a right coronary angiogram in the right anterior oblique projection.

Right Coronary Artery

A - Right Coronary Artery   F - Post. Descending Artery
B - SA Node Artery   G - AV Node Artery
C - Conus Artery   H - Septal Branches
D - Acute Marginal Artery   I - Postero Lateral Branches
E - Atrial Branch   K - Muscular Branches

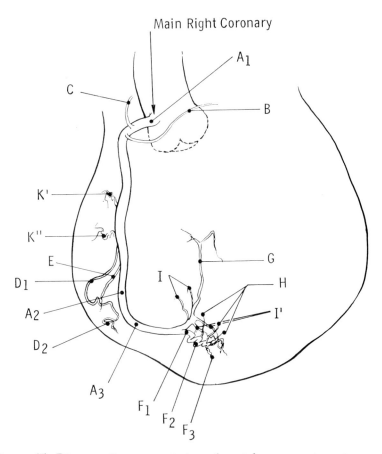

Figure 47. Diagramatic representation of a right coronary angiogram in the left anterior oblique projection (same patient as in Fig. 46).

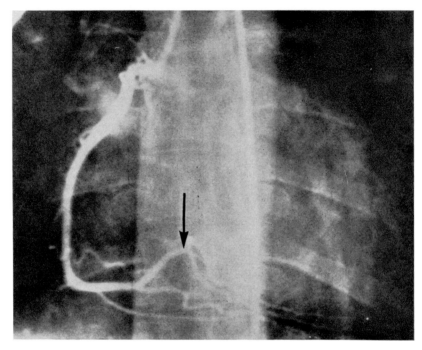

Figure 48. Antero-posterior projection of a selective right coronary angiogram. Note that the important vessels around the "crux" of the heart (arrow) cannot be well seen because they overlie the spine.

branch and ventricular branches are seen to travel towards the apex of the heart. On cine angiograms, they fold markedly during ventricular systole. The atrial branch, if it arises by itself, usually originates below the marginal branch. The distal right coronary artery, the U bend and the crux are not well seen in this projection. The posterior descending coronary artery, however, is well seen and runs towards the apex of the heart, sometimes meeting the distal portion of the anterior descending coronary artery. The posterolateral branches are somewhat parallel to the posterior descending coronary artery in this projection (see Fig. 55).

The RAO projection is most useful and should never be omitted. It will be noted that the right coronary artery is a very mobile structure and its motion has been compared to that of a

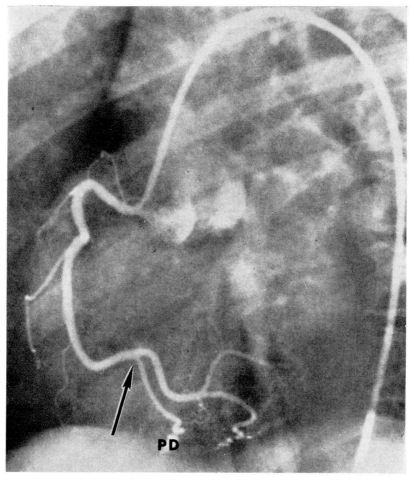

Figure 49. Left anterior oblique projection of a selective right coronary angiogram. Note that the posterior descending coronary artery does not originate at the crux but more proximally from the right coronary artery (see arrow).

windshield wiper. The "windshield wiper effect" is greatest in the RAO projection. Thus, radiographic films in this projection will often reveal motion if the exposure time has not been kept very short.

As already mentioned above, in the lateral projection, the right coronary artery should be posterior to the anterior de-

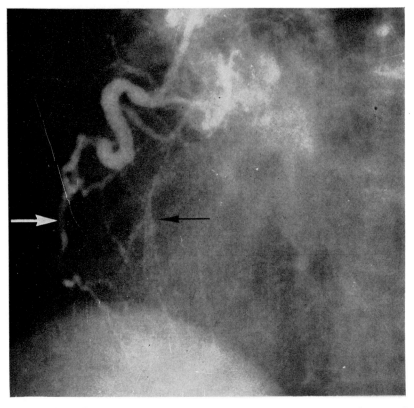

Figure 50. Selective right coronary arteriogram. Complete occlusion of the right coronary artery. In this projection one might mistake the marginal branch for the main right (see white arrow). Also note opacification of the left anterior descending coronary artery (black arrow).

scending coronary artery. If the right coronary is anterior this usually indicates right ventricular enlargement. The motion of the coronary arteries in this projection is minimized and overhead films usually are easily obtained. The posterior descending coronary artery, however, is not quite as well seen as in the RAO projection.

In the AP projection, the right coronary artery also demonstrates the same amount of motion as on the RAO projection. It usually overlies the spine and therefore this projection is not utilized.

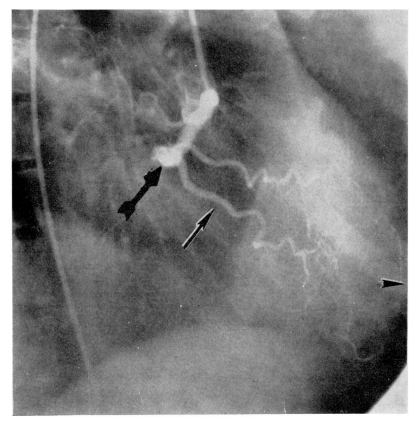

Figure 51. Right anterior oblique projection (same patient as Fig. 50). Note complete obstruction of the right (black arrow). The marginal branch seen in Figure 50 is here marked by a short black arrow. Arrowhead points to the left anterior descending coronary artery.

INTERCORONARY AND EXTRACORONARY ANASTOMOSIS

It has been shown that intercoronary anastomoses are numerous. The concept popularized by Cohnheim that coronary arteries are "end-arteries" has been disproven by Gross, Schlesinger, and many others.[5,6] Coronary angiography, however, is not sensitive enough to demonstrate these anastomoses under normal circumstances. These anastomoses only open when collateralization is necessary due to occlusion of a major vessel (this

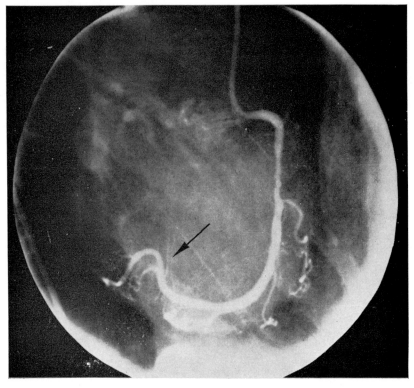

Figure 52. Lateral projection of a right coronary arteriogram. Note that there are two AV node arteries (black arrow).

is discussed in Chap. VIII). Extracoronary anastomoses have also been described. Thus the injection of anatomic specimens with dyes has shown flow from the coronary arteries to the vasa vasorum of the thoracic aorta and pulmonary artery as well as into the parietal pericardium, diaphragm and pleural surfaces of the lungs. Again, under normal circumstances, these vessels are not seen by coronary angiography and therefore will not be described here.

THE CARDIAC VEINS

The veins draining the cardiac capillary bed have a distribution which resembles that of the coronary arteries. Like all

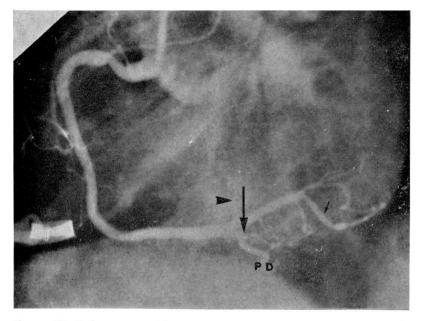

Figure 53. Left anterior oblique projection of a selective right coronary arteriogram. The narrowing seen proximally is caused by spasm (see Chap. X). Note that the posterior descending artery takes off classically at the crux of the heart (see black arrow), and is seen foreshortened. The posterolateral branches (short arrow) are parallel to the posterior descending artery. The AV node artery is marked by the arrowhead.

venous systems, these patterns may be variable; however, the main venous structures are fairly constant in their distribution.

The coronary veins are usually not opacified directly; instead, they are seen in the late phase of coronary angiography. As a rule the left coronary artery and its branches drain into the coronary sinus and therefore whenever the main left coronary artery is injected, the coronary sinus can be seen easily. Opacification of the right coronary artery often does not result in the visualization of the coronary sinus. The veins draining the right coronary arteries enter usually directly into the right atrium. However, if the distal right coronary artery provides a significant vascular supply to the left ventricle, the coronary sinus will then also be seen during the course of selective right coro-

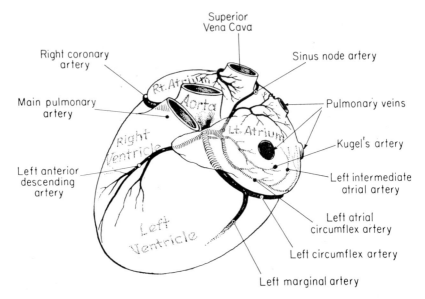

Superior
Vena Cava

Right coronary
artery

Sinus node artery

Main pulmonary
artery

Pulmonary veins

Kugel's artery

Left anterior
descending
artery

Left intermediate
atrial artery

Left atrial
circumflex artery

Left circumflex artery

Left marginal artery

Figure 54. Diagramatic representation of the course of the sinus node artery. The heart is viewed from above with the left ventricle facing the observer. Note that the sinus node artery turns around the superior vena cava. Adapted from Thomas N. James: *Anatomy of the Coronary Arteries.* Paul B. Hoeber, Inc., p. 127.

nary arteriography. In addition to the coronary sinus, smaller veins such as those draining into the coronary sinus can be opacified. One must not mistake such veins for arteries. When a major artery is occluded supply of blood to the distal portion of that vessel occurs through collaterals and is usually seen during the late angiographic phase. At times one may mistake a vein for a collateral channel which is opacifying later than the rest of the arteries.

ANATOMY

The coronary sinus enters the posterior wall of the right atrium. Its orifice is often guarded by a valve (Valve of Thebesius). This valve may prevent catheterization of the coronary sinus and is situated on the back of the right atrium. The coronary sinus itself extends towards the back of the left atrium

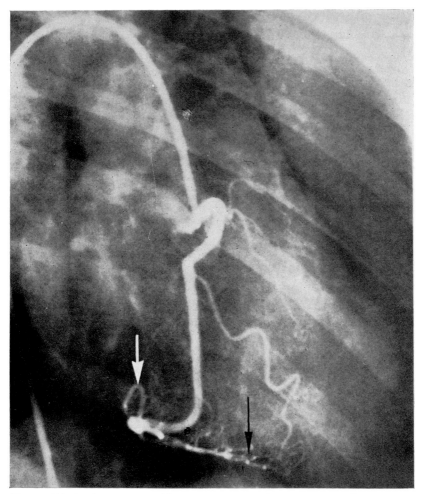

Figure 55. Right anterior oblique projection of a selective right coronary arteriogram. Figure 47 is the left anterior oblique projection of the same vessel. Note the U indicating the crux (short white arrow). The posterior descending artery (black arrow) can barely be separated from postero-lateral branches.

lying in the posterior AV groove. Its course roughly parallels that of the circumflex coronary artery.

The coronary sinus has three major tributaries. Those are the veins draining primarily the left ventricle, namely the anterior interventricular vein, the posterior interventricular vein, and the left marginal vein. Multiple names have been given to these veins and therefore the terminology is somewhat confusing.

1. The anterior interventricular vein, also called the great cardiac vein, begins at the apex of the heart and follows the anterior descending coronary artery in the anterior interventricular sulcus.

2. The posterior interventricular vein or middle cardiac vein begins near the apex of the heart posteriorly and runs in the posterior interventricular sulcus as does the posterior descending coronary artery.

3. The left marginal vein or posterior left ventricular vein runs on the diaphragmatic surface of the left ventricle accompanying branches of the left circumflex artery.

4. *Smaller Veins.* The oblique vein of the left atrium, also called oblique vein of Marshall, is a small vein which descends obliquely on the back of the left atrium. The anterior cardiac veins (3 or 4 in number) drain the ventral aspect of the right ventricle. All these veins usually connect with one another. The minimal cardiac veins of Thebesius are small venules which enter directly into the right atrium through orifices in the endocardial surface of that chamber. Occasionally during the injection of the right coronary artery, one might see these small structures.

REFERENCES

1. James, T.N.: *Anatomy of the Coronary Arteries.* New York, Paul B. Hoeber, Inc., 1961.
2. Bianchi, A.: Morfologia delle arteriae coronariae cordis. *Arch. Ital. Anat. e Embriol,* 3:87, 1904.
3. Schlesinger, M.J.: Relation of anatomic pattern to pathologic conditions of the coronary arteries. *Arch. Pathol.,* 30:403, 1940.
4. Schlesinger, M.J., Zoll, P.M., and Wessler, S.: The conus artery, a third coronary artery. *Am. Heart J.,* 38:823–836, 1941.
5. Gross, L.: *The Blood Supply to the Heart in its Anatomical and Clinical Aspects.* New York, Paul B. Hoeber, Inc., 1921.
6. Baroldi, G., Scomazzoni, G.: *Coronary Circulation in the Normal and Pathologic Heart.* Office of the Surgeon General, Dept. of the Army, Washington, D.C., 1967.

CHAPTER V

CONGENITAL ANOMALIES OF THE CORONARY VESSELS

To outline the coronary arterial patterns in congenital heart disease is of more than academic interest. Indeed, the surgeon may run into difficulty during corrective surgery if he is not forwarned of the presence of an unusual coronary artery pattern. In the early days of cardiac surgery, many a patient died because these anatomic variants were not appreciated. Although these patterns may be quite variable, there is a certain statistical likelihood of finding a given one for a given congenital heart disease. A review of these variants will be made. This discussion will be divided as suggested by Edwards[1] into anomalies of major significance (anomalies in which there is an abnormal communication between a coronary artery and a cardiac chamber or a major vessel other than another coronary artery) and anomalies of minor significance (those in which the coronary arteries arise entirely from the aorta, and present no hemodynamic burden for the patient).

ANOMALIES OF MAJOR SIGNIFICANCE

Anomalous Origin of the Coronary Arteries

Anomalous Origin of the Left Coronary Artery from the Pulmonary Artery

This condition is the most dramatic congenital anomaly of the coronary arteries and comes to the attention of the physician very early in the life of the patient. It is also the most common of the anomalous origins of the coronary arteries. In this condition, the left coronary artery arises either from the right but more often from the left pulmonary sinus (see Fig.

87

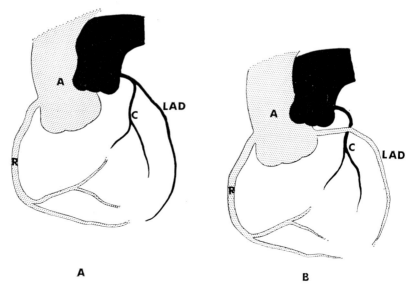

A   **B**

Figure 56. A, Diagramatic representation of the main left coronary artery arising from the left pulmonary sinus. B, Circumflex coronary artery arising from the left pulmonary sinus.

56A) but subsequently follows a normal course. The right coronary artery originates *normally* from the aorta. Blood flows from the right coronary artery to the left coronary artery in a retrograde manner and then fills the pulmonary artery (see Fig. 57A and B). The main resulting difficulty is not the left to right shunt, but the ischemia of the left ventricle. As a result, the left ventricular wall hypertrophies and fails to contract adequately. The papillary muscle ischemia produces dysfunction which in turn results in mitral insufficiency. This explains the appearance of the chest roentgenograms of these patients. The heart presents the features of a so-called "left sided obstructive lesion" with left ventricular and left atrial enlargement. The left atrial enlargement, however, is not as great as in endocardial fibroelastosis, and this may represent a distinguishing feature. Cases have also been described where the left anterior descending artery or the circumflex alone arises from the pulmonary artery (see Fig. 56B). These cases are rare. The resulting physiologic disturbances are identical to the one described above but usually better tolerated since a large portion of the left coronary artery arises normally.

Children affected by this condition come to the attention of the physician a few weeks after birth when the pulmonary resistance and, thus, the pulmonary artery pressure decrease sharply. As long as the pressure in the pulmonary artery is systemic (*in utero*) the perfusion of the left ventricle via the left coronary artery is adequate, but, when it drops, flow reversal occurs and severe ischemia may result. If collaterals between the right and left coronary arteries open up, the left ventricle is perfused via the right coronary artery. If, however, the collaterals are inadequate, severe ischemia will produce intractable left ventricular failure and result in early death. The electrocardiogram will demonstrate an infarction pattern with left ventricular hypertrophy and left ventricular strain. If the infant survives these first few weeks, his outlook is better, and he may live to adulthood. In fact, the first case, described by Abbott in 1908, was a sixty-year-old woman.[2] The definitive diagnosis is made by ascending aortography or, if the child is old enough, by selective coronary angiography (see Fig. 58). In all living cases, the right coronary artery is oversized, and delayed films demonstrate some opacification of the pulmonary artery via retrograde flow through the left coronary artery (see Fig. 57B). In spite of the left to right shunt, injection into the pulmonary artery may opacify the left coronary artery arising from it. This is explained by the pressure of the injection (see Fig. 59). The treatment was first suggested by Edwards,[3] who advised ligation of the left coronary artery at its origin from the pulmonary artery. This produces a flow pattern comparable to that of single coronary, which will be described subsequently in this chapter. This procedure prevents the rapid passage of blood from the left coronary artery into the pulmonary artery and gives the myocardium a greater chance to extract oxygen from the blood by which it is perfused. More recently, Armer devised a procedure by which the anomalous coronary is transplanted into the aorta.[4] To our knowledge, this procedure has not been very successful. However, with the present interest in coronary

artery surgery, a venous bypass combined with a proximal ligation of the left coronary artery should be technically feasible.

Anomalous Origin of the Right Coronary Artery from the Pulmonary Artery (Fig. 60B)

We have no experience with this lesion which seems to be
very rare. It was first described at autopsy by Brooks in 1866.[5]
The lesion is thought to be benign because the areas perfused
by the right coronary artery belong mostly to low pressure sys-

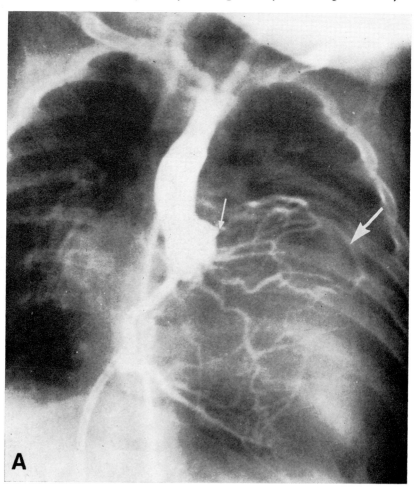

A

≫

tems (right ventricle and atrium). These chambers have a low systolic intramural tension and, therefore, can be supplied by a low pressure vessel. Thus, this condition is entirely compatible with life and is usually found at autopsy.

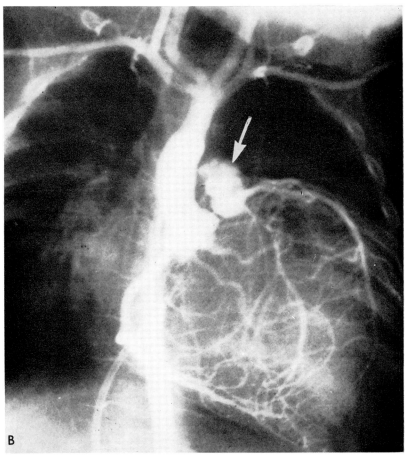

Figure 57. Aberrant left coronary artery arising from the pulmonary artery. A, Early phase of an ascending aortogram. Note that only a large right coronary arises from the aorta. There is a dimple (small arrow) where the left coronary artery should arise. The anterior descending coronary artery (large arrow) opacifies via collaterals. B, Later phase with opacification of the pulmonary artery indicating the left to right shunt. (arrow points to the opacified main pulmonary artery). From Baltaxe, H.A., *The Radiologic Clinics of North America*, Vol. IX, No. 3, Dec. 1971, pp. 597–607.

Anomalous Origin of Both Coronary Arteries from the Pulmonary Trunk (Fig. 60A)

Only a few cases of this anomaly have been reported in the literature. Tedeschi reviewed five cases from the World literature and found that only two cases, including his, had no other cardiac anomalies.[6] All infants died a few days after birth with the exception of one who died at age five months. Here again, we have no experience with this condition which, even if it were diagnosed early, would be most difficult to correct.

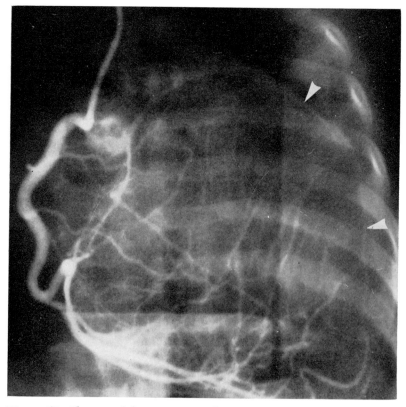

Figure 58. Aberrant left coronary. Selective right coronary arteriogram. Note the large number of collateral vessels allowing flow from right coronary artery to left coronary artery. Collateralization occurs mostly through the septum. White arrowheads point to left anterior descending coronary artery.

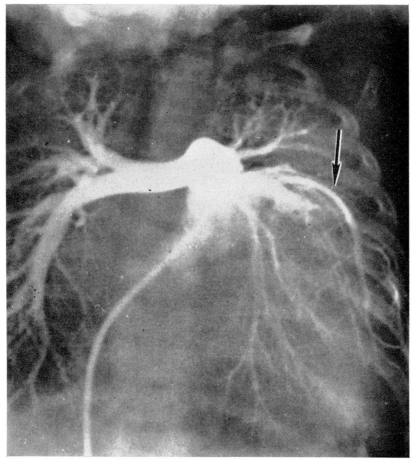

Figure 59. Pulmonary arteriogram. Same patient as Figure 57. Note the opacification of the left coronary artery (black arrow).

Coronary-Cardiac and Coronary Arteriorvenous Fistulae

By definition, a coronary-cardiac fistula is the connection of a coronary artery with one of the cardiac chambers. A coronary arteriovenous fistula is the connection of a coronary artery with a venous structure, usually the pulmonary artery or the coronary sinus.

In *coronary-cardiac fistulae*, the right coronary artery is more

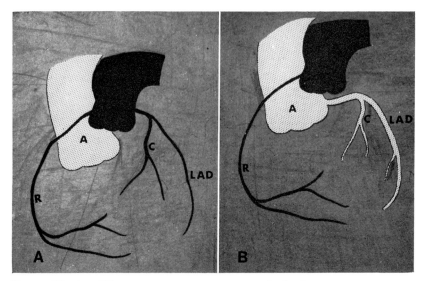

Figure 60. A, Diagramatic representation of both coronary arteries arising from the pulmonary artery. B, Right coronary artery arising from the pulmonary artery.

commonly involved and communicates, in decreasing order of frequency, with the right ventricle and the right atrium (see Fig. 61). When the left coronary artery is the site of involvement, the left main, the left anterior descending, or the left circumflex coronary arteries may communicate with the right ventricle, right atrium, or left ventricle (see Figs. 62 and 63).

In the coronary-cardiac fistulae, the artery communicating with a cardiac chamber is usually a large tortuous channel which may show one or more saccular aneurysms (see Fig. 61). It is often directly connected to the cardiac chamber but sometimes multiple small branches bridge the coronary artery and the cardiac cavity. These large arteries can produce a sizeable shunt. In such cases, the heart enlarges but for some unknown reason, the clinical picture remains relatively benign.

The *coronary arteriovenous fistulae* may develop between a branch of the left coronary artery and the main pulmonary artery. Fistulae between the right coronary artery and the pulmonary artery have also been described. In these shunts be-

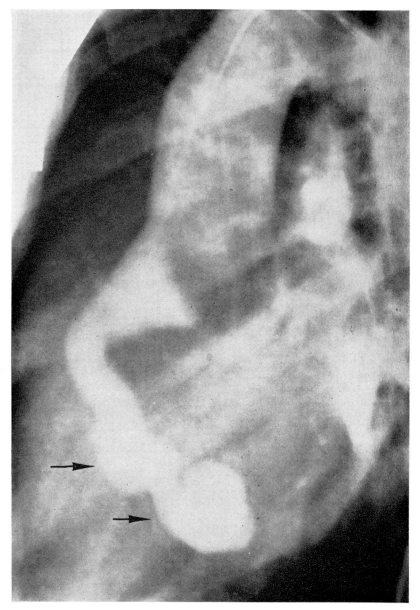

Figure 61. Right coronary to right atrium fistula. Note the tremendous enlargement of the right coronary artery and the formation of saccular aneurysms (arrows).

tween a coronary artery and a pulmonary artery, there are almost always multiple channels bridging the two structures, which makes surgery somewhat difficult (see Fig. 64). The fistulae represent a left to right shunt similar to that of a patent ductus arteriosus. The arteriovenous fistulae usually are rather small and may remain unnoticed until the patient develops coronary artery disease, at which time deprivation of oxy-

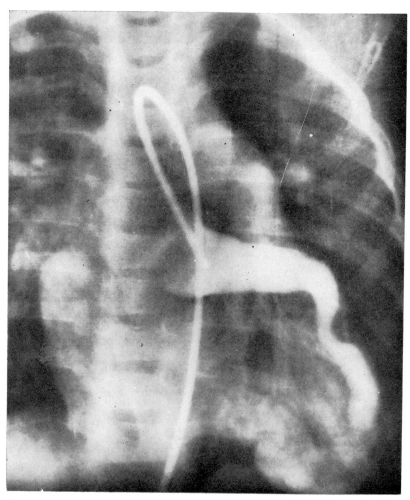

Figure 62. Left anterior descending coronary to left ventricle fistula. This is a selective injection into a markedly enlarged LAD.

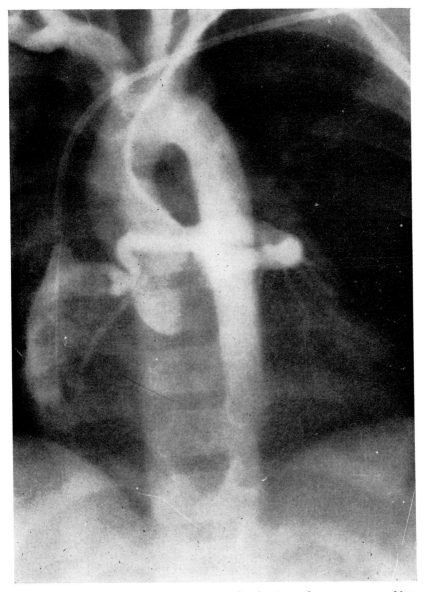

Figure 63. Left coronary to right atrium fistula. Ascending aortogram. Note the large channel arising from the left anterior descending coronary artery and ending in the right atrium. (This case was given to us by Dr. Murray Baron, Mount Sinai Hospital, New York City).

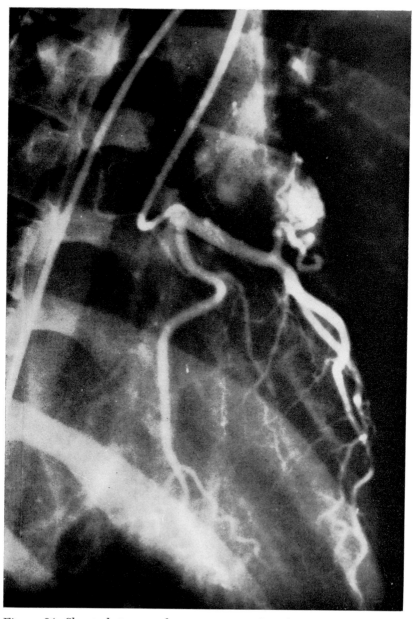

Figure 64. Shunt between the coronary and pulmonary artery with normal origin of the coronary arteries. Note the multiple small channels connecting the left anterior descending coronary artery to the pulmonary artery. This shunt represents no physiologic burden and is usually diagnosed because of a to and fro murmur. (Reproduced by permission from Gobel, *et al.: The American Journal of Cardiology,* 25:655–61, June 1970.)

gen and blood becomes a problem to an already ischemic myocardium. In our experience, however, most cases were asymptomatic and were detected during routine physical examinations.[7]

Surgery for both types of fistulae is performed to prevent a burden when atherosclerosis develops and to avoid bacterial endocarditis.[8] Furthermore, these large, tortuous vessels may be affected by thromboembolic complications. The operation consists of ligation of these vessels, which is usually a relatively benign procedure.

ANOMALIES OF MINOR SIGNIFICANCE

Anomalous Coronary Artery Patterns in Congenital Heart Disease

Predictable patterns exist in Tetralogy of Fallot and transposition complexes.

Tetralogy of Fallot

The most common pattern is the normal distribution. Lurie[14] describes four relatively frequent anatomic variants in Tetralogy of Fallot. The most frequent one is a large conal branch which arises from the right coronary artery and courses over the infundibulum of the right ventricle (see Type I, Fig. 65). This vessel must not be injured during ventriculotomy.

Secondly, a single right coronary artery has also been described in Tetralogy of Fallot. Usually a branch having the distribution of a left coronary artery arises from the right and courses in front of the pulmonary artery (see Type II, Fig. 65). Single left coronary arteries arising from the left coronary sinus have also been reported recently[15] (see Fig. 66).

Thirdly, the left coronary artery, instead of dividing early into circumflex and anterior descending branches, may course anteriorly and swing around the pulmonary artery. Only then does it divide into circumflex and anterior descending coronary arteries (see Type III, Fig. 65).

Fourthly, the anterior descending coronary artery arises from the right coronary artery and swings anteriorly to the pulmonary artery to reach the anterior interventricular groove. The circumflex artery arises normally from the left aortic sinus (Type IV, Fig. 65).

Transposition Complexes

Four types of transpositions will be considered:
1. Complete Transposition of the Great Vessels,
2. Corrected Transposition,

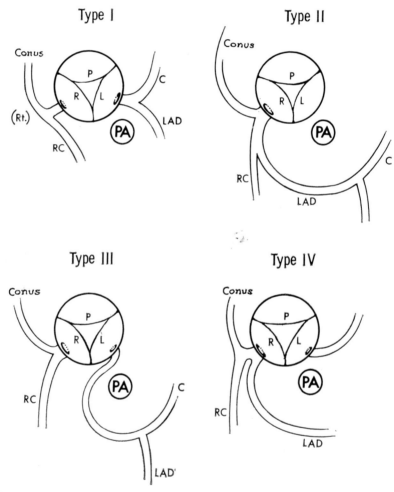

Figure 65. Diagramatic representation of the most common coronary patterns found in Tetralogy of Fallot.

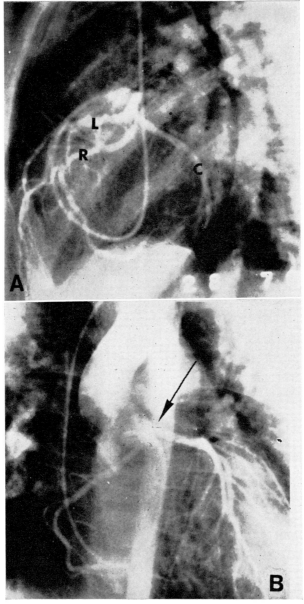

Figure 66. Single coronary artery arising from the left sinus of Valsalva (black arrow). The right coronary (R) is a branch of the left. A, Lateral projection (L = LAD, R = right coronary, C = circumflex). B. Antero-posterior aortogram. (Reproduced by permission from White, *et al.: American Journal of Roentgenology, 114/2:*350–54, Feb. 1972.)

3. Incomplete Transposition or Double Outlet Right Ventricle, and

4. Single Ventricle with Transposition of the Great Vessels. The above malformations will not be defined here as it is not in the scope of this book.

1. Transposition of the Great Vessels. The patterns described are according to the work of Elliot *et al.* who studied 115 pathologic specimens and seventeen live cases by angiography.[16] In complete transposition, the position of the right and noncoronary sinus is reversed. Three main patterns are found. In the first (see Type I, Fig. 67), the left coronary artery arises normally from the left sinus, divides as usual into anterior descending and circumflex coronary arteries, but is found anterior to the pulmonary artery (see Fig. 68).

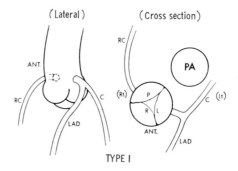

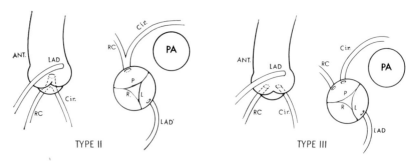

Figure 67. Diagramatic representation of the 3 most common coronary artery patterns found in transposition of the great vessels.

This of course is due to the nature of the transposition where the aorta is anterior to the pulmonary artery. Secondly (see Type II, Fig. 67), the left anterior descending artery arises from the left sinus but the circumflex artery originates from the right coronary artery (see Fig. 69) and courses behind the pulmonary artery to reach the left atrioventricular groove. Finally (see Type III, Fig. 67), the circumflex artery might arise by itself from the posterior sinus but still has the same course as described above. In those cases, the right coronary artery arises also from the posterior sinus but the left anterior descending arises from the left sinus (see Fig. 70).

Other less common patterns may be found and for further information the reader is referred to the classical paper of Elliot *et al.*

2. CORRECTED TRANSPOSITION. In this condition, the orientation of the aortic cusps is somewhat different from the normal one. There is an anterior cusp which is usually oversized and a right and left posterior cusp. Again there may be variations. We are describing the most common pattern.

The right coronary artery arises from the right sinus and divides immediately into a right and a left anterior descending coronary artery. The left circumflex artery, on the other hand, usually arises alone from the left aortic sinus and takes its normal course (see Figs. 71 and 72).

3. DOUBLE OUTLET RIGHT VENTRICLE. In this condition, both great vessels originate from the right ventricle and admixture of oxygenated and nonoxygenated blood occurs because of the presence of a ventricular septal defect which connects right and left ventricles.

Elliot *et al.*[16] reviewed fourteen cases of incomplete transposition but did not find a given anatomic pattern for the course of the coronary arteries. In fact, in most instances, the pattern was normal.

4. SINGLE VENTRICLE. By definition, a single ventricle is a condition in which both AV valves empty into the same chamber which thus receives the blood from both atria. This malformation is almost always associated with complete or corrected transposition of the great vessels. As a rule, the aorta arises from the

infundibulum whereas the pulmonary trunk is connected directly to the common ventricular chamber. In the presence of corrected transposition, the coronary artery pattern is as described under the heading "Corrected Transposition" (section 2). If complete transposition is present, the pattern is as described in section 1.

The general patterns described above are probably an over-simplification of the anatomic pattern which may be present in a given case. One should remember, however, that in the majority of cases the aforementioned patterns will be found and that only in rare instances will there be exceptions to these rules.

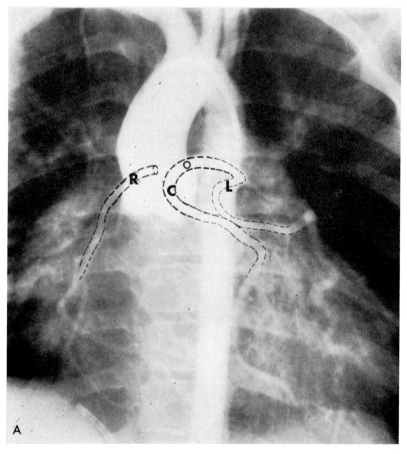

≫

Anomalous Origins of Coronary Arteries in Patients Usually Without Congenital Heart Disease

Single Coronary Artery

In cases of a single coronary artery, oxygenation of the myocardium occurs via only one vessel which arises from an ar-

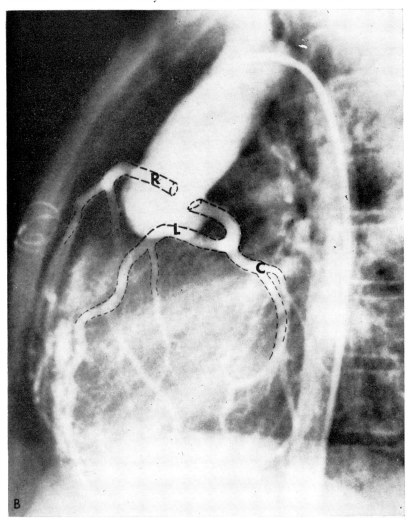

Figure 68. Transposition of great vessels. Type I coronary pattern. A, Antero-posterior projection of an ascending aortogram. B, Lateral projection (R = right coronary artery, L = LAD, C = circumflex).

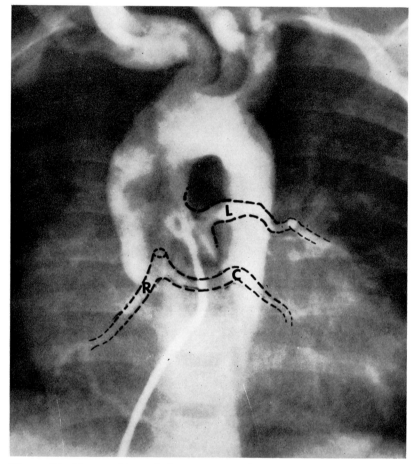

Figure 69. Transposition of the great vessels. Type II coronary pattern. Ascending aortogram in the antero-posterior projection. Same symbols as Figure 68.

terial trunk. This single vessel usually arises from the ascending aorta (see Fig. 66); however, cases have been reported in which it originated from the carotid artery and from the descending aorta.[9,10] These exceptions are extremely rare.

Single coronary artery is perfectly compatible with a normal life span. The oldest reported case died at age eighty after an abdominal peroneal resection of an adenocarcinoma of the rectum. The condition was first described by Thebesius in 1716.[11] Smith reviewed forty-five cases published in the World literature and divided them into three types.[12] In the first type, a single vessel follows the course of the normal right or left coronary artery, and thus supplies the territory of the absent vessel. For example, one may have an absent right coronary artery, but the circumflex is oversized and extends all the way over to the right anterior atrioventricular groove, giving rise to the posterior descending coronary artery. In those cases, there is a dimple in the right aortic sinus where the right coronary artery is supposed to originate.

In the second type, a single right or left coronary artery divides early and gives rise to a branch which is for all practical purposes the missing artery. We have seen cases in which the left coronary artery is absent with the right coronary artery giving off a branch which courses behind the aorta and then divides into the anterior descending and circumflex arteries.

Edwards[13] also describes a similar pattern in which the right coronary artery trifurcates and gives rise to a normal right coronary artery which runs in the right anterior atrioventricular groove, to a circumflex artery which passes posteriorly to reach the left posterior atrioventricular groove, and an anterior descending coronary which runs between the aorta and the pulmonary artery and reaches the anterior interventricular groove. When the right coronary artery is absent, an anomalous branch may originate from the main left coronary artery and may cross the pulmonary infundibulum in order to reach the right anterior atrioventricular groove.

The third type is usually associated with other cardiac congenital anomalies. In this group, the distribution of the single vessel is so atypical that no right or left pattern can be identified. Most of these patients in Smith's review died at an early age.

There is no sex predilection to this condition. The patients may reach adulthood, particularly when affected by the first and second type, but yet one-third of them die of cardiac disease. Bacterial endocarditis and myocardial infarction seem to represent the greatest danger in such individuals.

Other Forms of Coronary Ectopias

Ectopic origins of coronary arteries in patients with no congenital heart disease are found with relative frequency. Savolaire[17] found thirteen ectopic major coronary arteries in 1200
selective coronary arteriograms. All possible combinations of
coronary artery patterns have been described.

The right coronary artery presents less variations in origin
than the left. However, cases of right coronary arteries arising
from the left sinus of Valsalva have been reported. The right

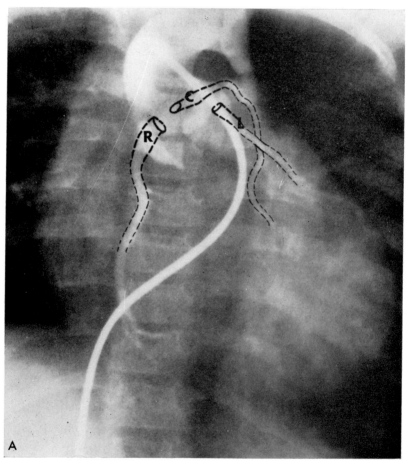

A

coronary artery may also be a branch of the circumflex artery which arises normally from the left.

Ectopia more commonly affects the left coronary artery. The left anterior descending and circumflex may arise from the left

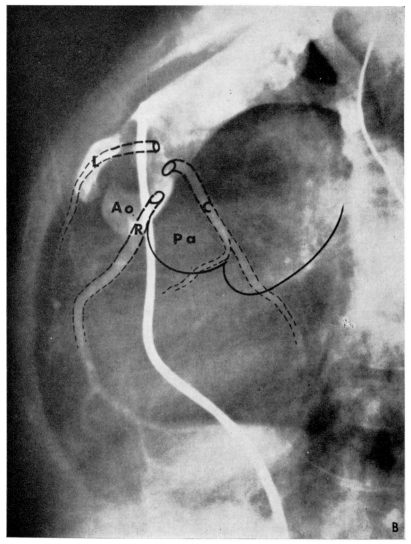

Figure 70. Transposition of the great vessels. Type III coronary artery pattern. A, Antero-posterior projection of an ascending aortogram. B, Lateral projection. Same code as Figure 68, Ao = aorta, Pa = pulmonary artery. Note the course of the catheter typical for T.G.V.

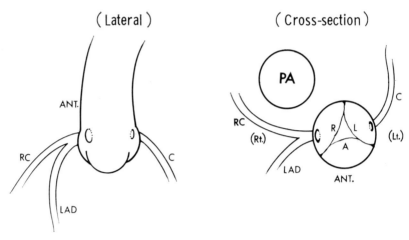

Figure 71. Corrected transposition. Coronary artery pattern. Diagramatic representation.

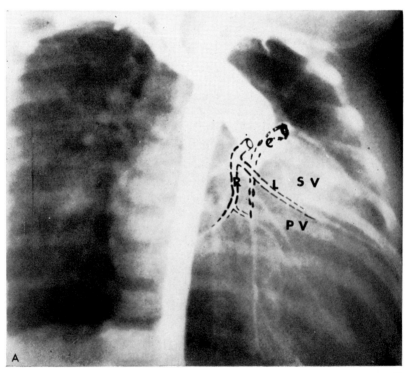

sinus from different ostia. The main left coronary artery may arise from the right sinus of Valsalva and later divide into left anterior descending and circumflex arteries. In our material, we found one case of left anterior descending and circumflex coronary arteries, each arising separately from the right sinus (see Fig. 73 and 74). Cases of the circumflex artery arising from the right coronary artery are relatively frequent (see Fig. 75 and 76). In those cases, the left anterior descending coronary artery arises normally from the left sinus.

It is conceivable that the left anterior descending coronary

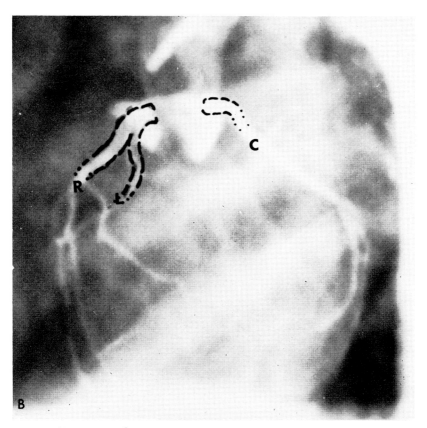

Figure 72. Corrected transposition. A, Antero-posterior projection of an ascending aortogram. B, Lateral projection (same code as Fig. 68) SV = systemic ventricle and PV = pulmonic ventricle.

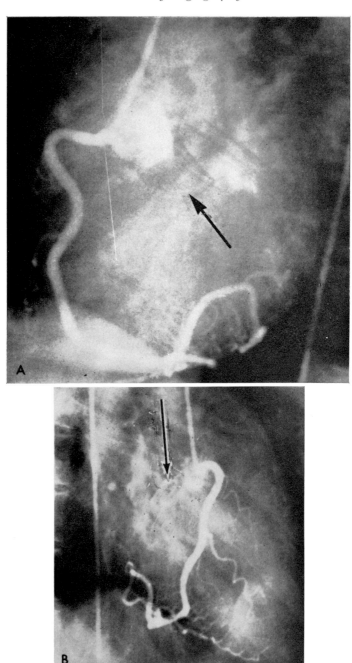

Figure 73. Selective right coronary arteriogram. A, Left anterior oblique projection. B, Right anterior oblique projection. Note flash filling of the circumflex artery (arrow) which has a separate orifice close to that of the right coronary artery.

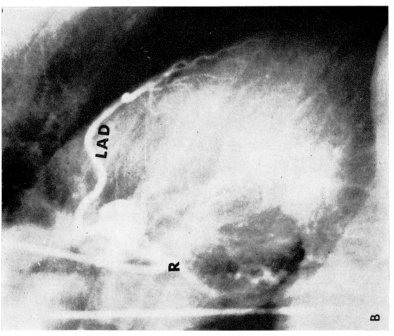

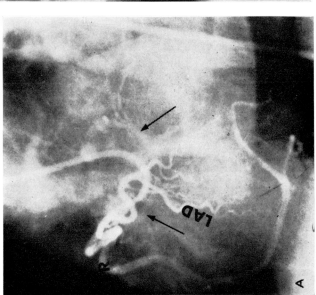

Figure 74. Selective left anterior descending coronary arteriogram. Note the position of catheter pointing to the right sinus of Valsalva. A, Left anterior oblique projection. B, Right anterior oblique projection. Note flash filling of the right and circumflex coronary arteries (arrows point to the circumflex coronary artery). Right, circumflex and LAD all arise from the right sinus from separate orifices.

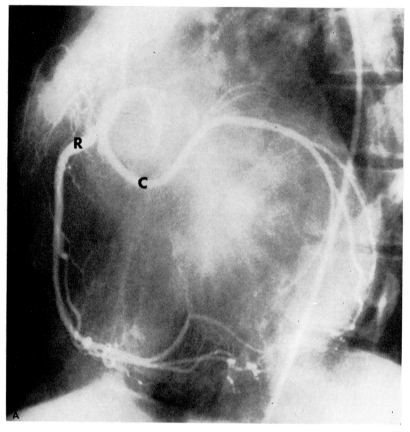

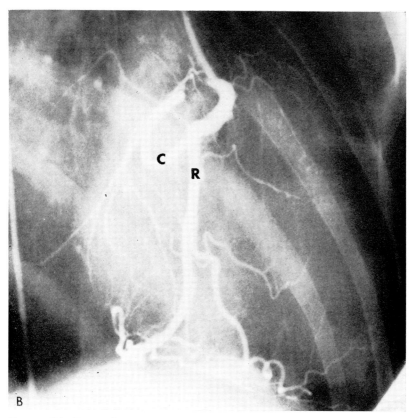

Figure 75. Circumflex coronary artery arising from the right coronary artery. Selective right coronary arteriogram. A, Left anterior oblique projection and B, Right anterior oblique projection.

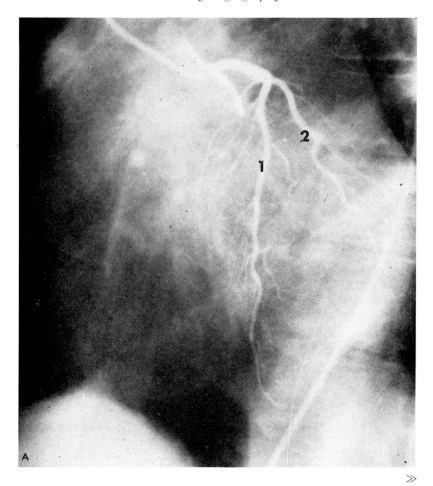

>>

artery may arise as a branch of the right coronary artery and that the circumflex originates normally from the left sinus.

Although this latter group of anomalies has no physiologic significance, it is important to be aware of these patterns. Indeed, during selective coronary angiography such patterns may represent a challenge for the angiographer. If a major branch of the coronary artery tree has not been opacified, one should rule out the possibility of ectopia by performing an ascending aortogram.

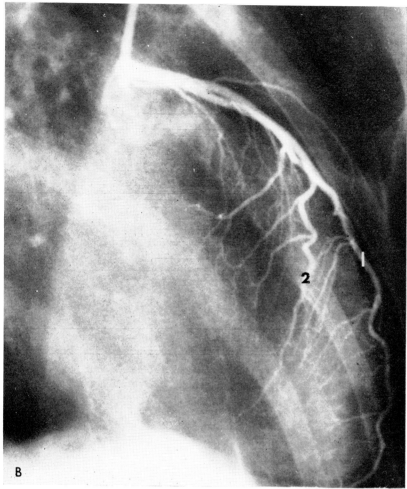

Figure 76. Same patient as in Figure 75. Selective anterior descending coronary arteriogram. Note the absence of a circumflex coronary artery. A, Left anterior oblique projection. B, Right anterior oblique projection. 1. LAD. 2. Diagnoal branch.

REFERENCES

1. Edwards, J.E.: Anomalous coronary arteries with special reference to arteriovenous like communications. *Circulation,* *14:*1001–1006, June, 1958.

2. Abbott, M.E.: *Congenital Cardiac Disease, in Osler's Modern Medicine.* Vol. 4, p. 420, Philadelphia, Lea and Febiger, 1908.

3. Edwards, J.E.: Functional pathology of congenital cardiac disease. *Pediat. Clin. N. Am., 1:*13, 1954.

4. Armer, R.M., Shumacker, H.B., Jr., Curie, P.R., and Fisch, C.: Origin of the left coronary artery from the pulmonary artery without collateral circulation. Report of a case with a suggested surgical correction. *Pediatrics, 32:*588, 1963.

5. Brooks, H. St. J.: Two cases of abnormal coronary artery of the heart arising from the pulmonary artery. *J. Anat. Physiol., 20:*26, 1866.

6. Tedeschi, C.G. and Helpern, M.M.: Heterotopic origin of both coronary arteries from the pulmonary artery. Review of literature and report of a case not complicated by associated defects. *Pediatrics 14:*53–57, 1954.

7. Gobel, F.L., Anderson, C.F., Baltaxe, H.A., Amplatz, K., and Wang Yang: Shunts between the coronary and pulmonary arteries with normal origin of the coronary arteries. *Am. J. Cardiol., 25:*655–661, June 1970.

8. Effler, D.B., Sheldon, W.C., Turner, J.J., and Groves, L.K.: Coronary arteriovenous fistulas: Diagnosis and surgical management. Report of fifteen cases. *Surgery, 61/1:*41–50, Jan. 1967.

9. Bjork, V.O. and Bjork, K.L.: Coronary artery fistula. *J. Thorac. Cardiovasc. Surg., 49/6:*921–930, June 1965.

10. Edwards, J.E.: *Atlas of Congenital Anomalies.* Springfield, Ill., Thomas, 1954.

11. Thebesius, A.C.: Dissestatio Medica de Circulo Sanguinis in Cordo Ludg. Batav, J.A. Langerack, 1716.

12. Smith, J.C.: Review of single coronary artery with report of 2 cases. *Circulation, 1:*1168, 1950.

13. Edwards, J.E.: Congenital malformations. F. Malformations of the coronary vessels. In *Pathology of the Heart,* S.E. Gould (Ed.). Springfield, Ill., Thomas, pp. 425–34.

14. Lurie, P.R.: Abnormalities and Diseases of the Coronary Vessels in Heart Disease in Infants, Children and Adolescents. Moss and Adams (Eds.). Baltimore, Williams and Wilkins Co., pp. 738–759.

15. White, R.I., Frech, R.S., Castaneda, A., and Amplatz, K.: The nature and significance of anomalous coronary arteries in Tetralogy of Fallot. *Am. J. Roentgenol., 114/2:*350–54, Feb. 1972.

16. Elliot, L.P., Amplatz, K., Edwards, J.E.: Coronary arterial patterns in transposition complexes. Anatomic and angiographic studies. *Am. J. Cardiol., 17:*362–78, March 1966.

17. Savolaire, E.R. and Molnar, W.: Ectopic origin of coronary arteries in non-congenital heart disease based on 1200 selective coronary studies. Read to the 57th Scientific Assembly and Annual Meeting. The Radiological Society of North America, Nov. 28, 1971.

CHAPTER VI

COMPLICATIONS—CONTRAINDICATIONS— INDICATIONS

COMPLICATIONS

It is appropriate to precede a discussion of the indications for a procedure by a section describing its complications. The decision to perform coronary angiography should be influenced by the complication rate in a given hospital. When discussing complication rates, most authors refer to Ross and Gorlin's study[4] of 3312 coronary arteriograms. Lately, however, more data have become available.[2,5,11,17]

The complications usually reported are as follow:

1. *Myocardial Infarction* can occur during or within a few hours after coronary angiography. It may be caused by the injection of a clot, air (see Fig. 77), or fibrin into the coronary arteries.[1,2] Dissection of the vessel by the tip of the catheter may produce a massive infarction with or without instantaneous death.[3] Embolization produced by the dislodgment of an atherosclerotic plaque in the course of the manipulation of the catheter is also possible. Sones admits to myocardial infarction in only 0.3 per cent of cases whereas most other investigators report a frequency of at least 0.9 per cent.[4] Recently a large center[5] reported a frequency of 2.6 per cent of nonfatal myocardial infarctions in five hundred patients.

In order to minimize the rate of complications, the catheter must be flushed frequently. This is always important but particularly when one utilizes polyurethane material. Recently, scanning electron microscopy has shown that polyurethane has greater surface roughness than polyethylene.[6] Nachnani et al.[6] have shown that physical surface defects are important factors in the initiation of thrombogenesis on vascular catheter

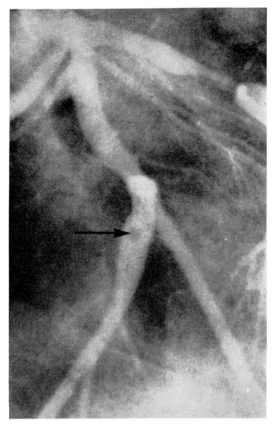

Figure 77. Injection of an air bubble (see arrow) into the circumflex coronary artery. Note the severe narrowing of the left anterior descending coronary artery.

surfaces. In light of these findings, we have switched to polyethylene catheters and our initial impression is that the rate of complication has decreased. The addition of Heparin to the flushing solution may also be helpful. Newer developments such as Heparin binding to plastic catheters may significantly reduce the incidence of catheter thrombogenesis.[7] The Teflon coated guide wires must be cleaned thoroughly as their surfaces often accumulate clots which may be stripped off during catheter insertion.[2]

Dissection of the wall of the coronary arteries is difficult to avoid. The left "Judkins" catheter for instance has a tendency to spring rapidly into the lumen of the left coronary artery when it is advanced within the ascending aorta after the guide wire is removed. This sudden springing of the catheter tip may dissect, occlude or perforate[8] the lumen of the artery and result in the death of the patient. On rare occasions, dissection has also occurred with the right Judkins or Amplatz coronary catheters as well as with the Sones catheter. Only very gentle manipulation of the catheter during its introduction into the coronary ostium will avoid this complication. The bullet-nose catheter tip is supposed to prevent dissection but does not always succeed in its mission. If dissection has occurred, it is of utmost importance that the angiographer be aware of it immediately in order not to inject flushing solution or contrast and thereby extend the dissection. Therefore, continuous pressure monitoring during the catheterization is important. No injection should be performed unless an adequate pressure tracing is read on the monitor. Failure to obey this rule may lead to further dissection of the artery during the injection of solution and produce instantaneous death. It is conceivable that if a localized dissection is identified and the procedure discontinued, the subintimal hematoma might resorb and the patient survive without complications. In young patients without coronary artery disease, a dissection can be fairly well tolerated. We have witnessed two dissections which did not produce myocardial damage (see Fig. 78). On the other hand, the presence of a normal pressure reading does not guarantee that the catheter tip is not subintimal.

In patients with severe coronary artery disease, the hypoxia produced by the contrast agent may alone precipitate myocardial infarction. No definitive work has yet been done on the effect of contrast media upon the myocardium during coronary angiography. Hypotension caused by the injection of contrast or by the administration of nitroglycerin may suffice to precipitate a myocardial infarction.

2. *Arrythmias* developed in twenty-seven patients in Ross' series[4] of 3264 (forty-eight patients had more than one pro-

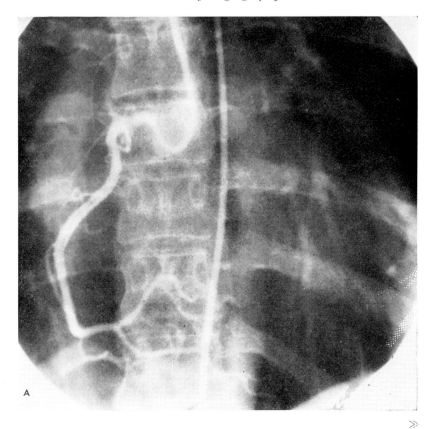

A

cedure). Of these, twenty-four patients developed ventricular fibrillation, an incidence of 0.75 per cent. It occurred in thirteen patients where Hypaque M 75%[*] was injected and in six where Renovist[†] was used. These patients were defibrillated electrically and recovered. In our experience with Renografin 76,[†] ventricular fibrillation due to the contrast is extremely rare and has not occurred in the last 750 cases. Judkins reports an absence of contrast-induced ventricular fibrillation in over 3000 selective coronary injections.[9] Renografin 76 contains 0.19 mEq. of sodium/cubic centimeter. This appears to be just the proper amount for safe use. In 1970, when the manufacturer changed

[*] Made by Winthrop.
[†] Made by Squibb.

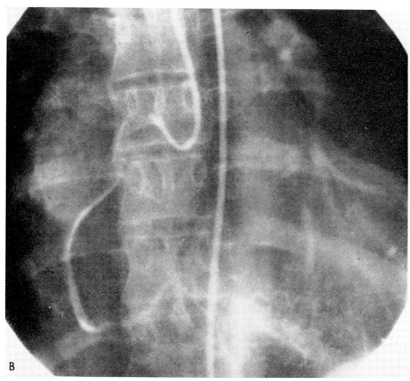

B

Figure 78. Dissected right coronary artery. A, Selective right coronary arteriogram. Note the lucent defect within the vessel representing intima. B, Late arterial phase. Contrast in subintimal position does not wash out.

the composition of Renografin 76 by removing most of the sodium,* a high incidence of ventricular fibrillation ensued. They, therefore, reverted to the original formula. Contrast media which have either a much higher or lower sodium concentration tend to produce ventricular fibrillation.

Asystole occurred twice (Ross' series) immediately after the injection of contrast material. Both patients received closed chest massage and recovered. A third patient developed asystole fifteen minutes after the procedure and died. In our experience, asystole lasting more than fifteen seconds has not been a problem. Green *et al.* reported one death in 445 examinations due to "bradyarrythmia."[2]

* Now this contrast material is called Reno-M-60 or 76.

3. There were *three deaths* in Ross' series of 3,312 coronary arteriography procedures. Sones reports twelve deaths in 13,602 patients (0.09%).[10] Of those, three had a dissection of the right coronary artery. Dissection of the left coronary is more common with the femoral approach. Judkins claims a mortality rate of two in 4,500 patients.[9] Some have tried to relate a greater complication rate to the technique utilized. However, with a greater number of centers performing the procedure, it has become apparent that the complication rate varies considerably from center to center. Data gathered in San Francisco,[11] for instance, showed that mortality may be related to the number of cases performed in a given hospital. At six hospitals, the mortality varied from 0.5 per cent among 650 cases to 8 per cent among twenty-five cases with an overall mortality of 1 per cent among 2,025 cases. In addition to the experience of the team, patient selection is also important. Large referral centers often examine a type of patient who is ambulatory, able to travel long distances, and whose disease is not as severe as that of patients seen in smaller centers.

4. *Among the noncardiac complications,* thrombosis of the catheterized femoral or brachial artery is the most common. Femoral artery thrombosis occurs in roughly 1 per cent of the cases.[12-14] It is important that the operator recognize this complication even prior to withdrawing his arterial catheter. It is customary in our laboratory to inject contrast material into the iliac artery through the catheter that has been used for angiography when pulsations of the dorsalis pedis or posterior tibial artery cannot be felt at the end of the procedure (assuming it was present at the beginning). This will allow angiographic localization of the site of thrombosis. In those cases, rapid removal of a clot is usually performed by the surgeon under local anesthesia. Thrombosis of the brachial artery was reported by some in 0.3 per cent of cases; however, a rate of 0.4 to 1.4 per cent is more realistic.[15] Surgical exposure of the brachial artery has the advantage of allowing removal of thrombi prior to repair of the catheterized arteries. It is now customary in Sones' laboratory to inflate the balloon of a Fogerty catheter in the innominate artery and pull it back, thus removing thrombi

which form on the outside of the catheter and which might cause brachial artery thrombosis. This procedure apparently has significantly reduced the incidence of post-catheterization thrombosis of the brachial artery.

In the case of post-catheterization thrombosis, it has to be emphasized that occlusion of the brachial artery may be well tolerated and without clinical consequences. On the other hand, post-catheterization thrombosis of the femoral artery invariably results in arterial insufficiency and requires surgical thrombectomy. Even if signs of ischemia may be absent at rest, they will appear at the time of exercise if a thrombus has not been removed.

Embolization of clots originating from the inner or outer surface of the catheter may produce strokes (0.8% of 500 cases),[5] renal and mesenteric infarctions, or occlusion of distal vessels in the legs.

Allergic reactions to the contrast material are rare in our experience, and are confined to urticarial skin lesions. Anaphylactic shock has not occurred in our laboratories.

Large hematomas at the puncture site may have to be evacuated and could get infected. If the arterial puncture was done above the inguinal ligament, bleeding into the pelvis might be more difficult to control. Delayed bleeding was reported to occur eight to twelve hours after termination of the procedure in nine patients among 445.[2]

Post-catheterization fevers are not rare and could be due to pyrogenic reactions or to bacteremia caused by poor sterile technique. Patients with fever are usually rapidly treated with antibiotics and suffer no after-effects. Infections may delay surgery and could cause prolonged hospitalization. Meticulous sterile technique should be utilized in order to avoid this complication.

CONTRAINDICATIONS

It is generally felt that coronary angiography should not be performed within one month of an acute myocardial infarction. The usual reason given is that shortly after an infarction the myocardium is more irritable. Thus, the intracoronary injection of contrast medium might result in severe arrythmias.

In the presence of acute congestive heart failure or impending failure, contrast material injected into the coronary arteries may be dangerous. It is well known that the injection of contrast agents into the left ventricle, as well as into the coronary arteries, produces an elevation of the ventricular end diastolic pressure.[16] This elevation seems to be more severe when the myocardium is damaged and therefore coronary angiography could produce pulmonary edema.

Arrhythmias of all types should be carefully evaluated prior to angiography and the procedure should be postponed until a stable state has been reached; this is particularly true for digitalis toxicity.

Hypokalemia should be corrected prior to angiography as it may cause ventricular fibrillation during the procedure. The blood potassium level should be 4 mg % or above.

INDICATIONS

The indications for coronary angiography have become broader as surgery has markedly widened its scope.[17,18] For the sake of simplicity, the indications will be broken down into several groups of patients in the following fashion:

1. Those suffering from angina.
2. Those not suffering from angina.

Patients with Angina

Angina is not always easy to diagnose and lesions such as cervical osteoarthritis, hiatus hernia, intercostal neuritis, cholecystitis, and peptic ulcer must be ruled out prior to submitting someone to coronary angiography. Amongst patients who have angina, one finds those who have had one or several documented myocardial infarctions and those without known previous infarction.

Patients with a History of Infarction

Patients who have had a well-documented myocardial infarction and who still suffer from angina obviously need help.

It is now believed by many that if these patients do not respond to medical therapy, surgery might be beneficial. The reader must, however, realize that this topic is still very controversial. Some cardiologists are of the opinion that coronary arteriography and subsequent surgery should only be offered to those patients who are severely incapacitated, whereas others believe that coronary artery surgery might protect the patient with mild symptoms from future infarctions. In any event, coronary angiography should probably not be performed if surgery is not contemplated.

At present, patients in cardiogenic shock represent the only group who are treated surgically immediately following acute myocardial infarction.[19] Recently, several centers have performed angiography and operated successfully upon such patients[20] with the hope of preventing extension of the infarct and improving function of the remaining viable myocardium. This is considered a method of last resort, since cardiogenic shock carries an extremely high mortality on medical therapy alone. Circulatory assistance by means of an intra-aortic balloon pump might be necessary before and during coronary angiography.

Patients Without a Documented Myocardial Infarction

In recent years, more and more patients complaining of angina are referred for angiography, although they had no previous history of myocardial infarction. The majority of these patients have severe coronary artery disease but maintain good myocardial function, and sometimes have a normal electrocardiogram. At times, even stress electrocardiograms may remain negative in the presence of coronary artery disease. Thus, patients incapacitated by chest pain where noncardiac causes have been excluded, in spite of absence of a previous infarction, and even in the presence of a normal resting or exercise electrocardiogram, should be investigated by angiography.

A small number of these patients will have normal coronary arteries and the cause of their angina often cannot be explained. Occlusion of relatively small branches of major vessels,[21] small vessel disease, abnormal oxyhemoglobin dissociation,[22] and inadequate resolution of the radiographic methods have all been incriminated. It has been shown, however, that these patients have a near normal life expectancy and an excellent prognosis.[23]

Another group of patients in this category are those who have not had a previous infarction but who suddenly have developed chest pain and electrocardiographic changes typical of a preinfarction pattern. Coronary angiography in these patients is definitely more hazardous but justified if one believes that coronary artery surgery might prevent infarction.[20]

Aortic stenosis causes low cardiac output which might produce myocardial ischemia and therefore angina. Many believe that in the presence of aortic stenosis and angina, coronary angiography should be performed to rule out atherosclerotic involvement of the coronary arteries.

Patients Without Angina

Several groups are found without angina.

Patients with Previous Myocardial Infarction

It is believed in some centers that any patient under the age of fifty who has had a documented myocardial infarction should have coronary angiography even though he has no history of angina. The purpose of the study would be to define the extent of the disease and perhaps to perform "preventive" surgery. The value of the surgery is, however, questionable.

Patients Without a History of Myocardial Infarction but with Electrocardiographic Abnormalities

These patients are rather rare. We have seen a number of patients with no previous history of myocardial infarction or angina, exhibiting suspicious electrocardiographic changes during a yearly check-up. Among airline pilots and persons in other responsible positions, it may be quite important to determine whether coronary artery disease is present and the only definitive test is coronary angiography.

Chronic Heart Failure of Unknown Etiology

Patients with CHF who have not had a known myocardial infarction and who do not have angina, may have a myocardiopathy or coronary artery disease. Coronary angiography will help to separate the two entities, although it is conceivable that atherosclerosis and myopathy might be coexistant.

Preoperative Evaluation Prior to Valve Surgery

In cases of aortic stenosis, where the patient is complaining of angina, the symptomatology might be due either to insufficient perfusion of the coronary arteries or to coronary artery disease as discussed above. In those instances, coronary arteriography is indicated. Even when angina is absent, some surgeons today feel that if the patient is to have coronary artery perfusion during cardiac bypass, coronary arteriography should be obtained. Obviously, if a major branch of the left coronary artery is severely diseased, coronary artery perfusion is ineffective If a significant lesion is discovered on preoperative coronary angiography, some surgeons perform a saphenous venous bypass at the time of the replacement of the valve.

Congenital Heart Disease

Congenital anomalies of the coronary arteries have been discussed in Chapter V. The diagnosis of coronary artery fistulae and connections between the coronary and the pulmonary arteries can be best diagnosed by selective studies. When this diagnosis is seriously considered, selective coronary arteriography should be obtained.

Follow-up and Investigative Studies

In order to manage patients who have had bypass procedures, many surgeons feel that it is important to perform follow-up angiograms. The patients who have had saphenous venous bypasses are reinvestigated sometimes shortly after surgery and also on a yearly basis.[24] Since atherosclerosis is a progressive disease, reexamination of their coronary arteries should be performed at the same time.

An example of an investigative clinical study is that of Buchwald who treated patients with hypercholesteremia by resection of a large amount of bowel in order to prevent reabsorption of cholesterol at the level of the ileum. The effectiveness of this procedure has been evaluated by serial coronary angiograms which have shown that although atherosclerosis is progressive, it can be slowed down and sometimes arrested by the operation.[25]

On a more investigative basis, coronary flow studies have been performed by injecting Xenon 133 into the ostium of the coronary arteries.[26] Myocardial perfusion scans are performed by injecting $_{131}I$ macroaggregate particles during selective coronary angiography.[27]

REFERENCES

1. Lichtlen, P.: Complications of selective coronary arteriography. In Kaltenbach, M. and Lichtlen, P. (Eds.): *Coronary Heart Disease,* Stuttgart, Germany, Georg Thieme Verlag, 1971.
2. Green, G.S., McKinnon, M., Roesch, J., and Judkins, M.P.: Complications of selective percutaneous transfemoral coronary arteriography and their prevention. A review of 445 consecutive examinations. *Circulation, XLV:*553–57, 1972.
3. Haas, J.M., Peterson, C.R., and Jones, R.C.: Subintimal dissection of the coronary arteries. A complication of selective coronary arteriography and the transfemoral percutaneous approach. *Circulation, 38:* 678–683, 1968.
4. Ross, R.S. and Gorlin, R.: Coronary arteriography. *Circulation Supplement III,* Vols. 37 and 38, pp. 67–73, 1968.
5. Wexler, L.: Coronary arteriography: Complications and indications, questions and answers. *J.A.M.A.,* 219/7:917–18, 1972.
6. Nachnani, G.H., Lessin, L.S., Motomiya, T., and Jensen, W.N.: Scanning electron microscopy of thrombogenesis on vascular catheter surfaces. *New Engl. J. Med.,* 286/3:139–40, 1972.
7. Glancy, J.J., Fishbone, G., and Heinz, E.R.: Nonthrombogenic arterial catheters. *Am. J. Roentgen.,* 108:716, 1970.
8. Morethin, M.D. and Wallace, J.M.: Uneventful perforation of a coronary artery during selective arteriography. A case report. *Am. J. Roentgen.,* 110:184, 1970.

9. Judkins, M.P.: Personal communication.

10. Sones, F.M.: Cine coronary arteriography. *Anesth. Analg., 46:*499, 1967.

11. Selzer, A., Anderson, W.L., and March, H.W.: Indications for coronary arteriography: Risks *vs.* benefits. *Calif. Med., 115:*1–6, 1971.

12. Lang, E.K.: A survey of the complications of percutaneous retrograde arteriography. Seldinger technique. *Radiology, 81:*257, 1963.

13. Siegelman, S., Caplan, L.H., and Annes, G.P.: Complications of catheter angiography: Study with oscillometry and "pullout" angiograms. *Radiology, 91:*251, 1968.

14. Kloster, F.E., Bristow, J.D., Griswold, H.E.: Femoral artery occlusion following percutaneous catheterization. *Am. Heart J., 79:*175, 1970.

15. Campion, B.C., Frye, R.L., Pluth, J.R., Fairbairn, J.F., and Davis G.D.: Arterial complications of retrograde brachial arterial catheterization. *Mayo Clin. Proc., 46:*589, 1971.

16. Levin, D.C. and Baltaxe, H.A.: The effect of intracoronary and interventricular injection of radiopaque contrast material upon left ventricular end diastolic pressure (LVEDP). Exhibited at the Annual Meeting of the American Roentgen Ray Society, Sept. 20, 1971. *New York State Medical Jour.* 72:2619, 1972.

17. Takaro, T., Dart, C.H., Jr., Scott, S.M. *et al.:* Coronary arteriography: Indications, techniques, complications. *Ann. Thorac. Surg., 5:*213–221, 1968.

18. Ross, R.S.: Clinical applications of coronary arteriography. *Circulation,* 27:107–11, 1963.

19. Mundt, E.D., Yurchak, P.M., Buckley, M.J., Leinbach, R.C., Kantrowitz, A., and Austen, W.G.: Circulatory assistance and emergency direct coronary artery surgery for shock complicating acute myocardial infarction. *New Engl. J. Med., 283:*1382–84, 1970.

20. Scanlon, P..J., Nemickas, R., Tobin, J.R., Jr., Anderson, W., Montoya, A., Pifarre, R.: Myocardial revascularization during acute phase of myocardial infarction. *J.A.M.A., 218/2:*207–212, 1971.

21. James, T.M.: Angina without coronary disease (sic). *Circulation, 42:* 189–91, 1970.

22. Eliot, R.S. and Bratt, G.: The paradox of myocardial ischemia and necrosis in young women with normal coronary arteriograms: Relation to abnormal hemoglobin-oxygen dissociation. *Am. J. Cardiol.,* 23:633–38, 1969.

23. Waxler, E.B., Kimbiris, D., and Driefus, S.L.: The fate of women with normal coronary arteriograms and chest pain resembling angina pectoris. *Am. J. Cardiol., 28:*25–32, 1971.

24. Baltaxe, H.A., Carlson, R.G., and Lillehei, C.W.: Roentgenographic appearance of aorto-coronary artery bypass using a reversed saphenous vein. *Am. J. Roentgen., 60:*734–38, 1970.

Coronary Angiography

25. Baltaxe, H.A., Amplatz, K., Varco, R.L., Buchwald, H.: Coronary arteriography in hypercholesterolemic patients. *Am. J. Roentgen.*, *55*:786–90, 1969.
26. Baltaxe, H.A., Formanek, G., Loken, M., and Amplatz, K.: Clinical limitation to use of Xenon for measurement of myocardial blood flow. *Invest. Radiol.*, *4*:317–22, Sept-Oct, 1969.
27. Ashburn, W.L., Braunwald, E., Simon, A.L., Peterson, K.L., and Gault, J.H.: Myocardial perfusion imaging with radioactive-labeled particles injected directly into the coronary circulation of patients with coronary artery disease. *Circulation*, *44*:851–865, 1971.

CHAPTER VII

ELECTROCARDIOGRAPHIC AND HEMODYNAMIC CHANGES SEEN DURING SELECTIVE CORONARY ARTERIOGRAPHY

The injection of contrast material into the coronary artery produces electrocardiographic and hemodynamic changes which are characteristic for each coronary artery but which are not entirely understood. The description of these changes will be rather brief and we will limit ourselves to practical considerations. It is hoped that this chapter will help the angiographer to understand the changes occurring on the monitor during coronary arteriography.

ELECTROCARDIOGRAPHIC CHANGES

Typical Changes Involving the Left Coronary Artery (See Fig. 79)

The electrocardiographic changes for both coronary arteries differ with injections into normal and abnormal vessels. Some features, however, seem to be fairly constant.[1,2] During the injection into the left coronary artery standard leads 2 and 3 often show a decrease in the peak P wave amplitude, as well as a decrease in the height of the R wave and/or an increase in depth of the S wave. In addition, there is usually an increase in the QRS amplitude. The most characteristic change, however, is the increase in the mean T wave amplitude which occurs in 95 per cent of patients. The Q-T interval is prolonged and the heart rate is decreased.

With contrast injection into the left coronary artery, the QRS vector seems to shift counterclockwise to the left and the T wave vector shifts clockwise to the right.[3]

133

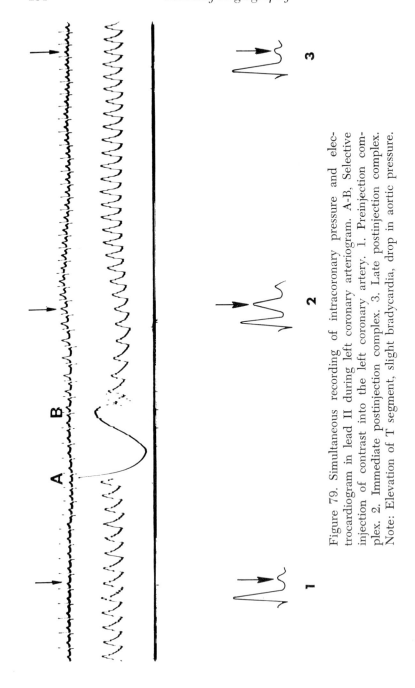

Figure 79. Simultaneous recording of intracoronary pressure and electrocardiogram in lead II during left coronary arteriogram. A-B, Selective injection of contrast into the left coronary artery. 1. Preinjection complex. 2. Immediate postinjection complex. 3. Late postinjection complex. Note: Elevation of T segment, slight bradycardia, drop in aortic pressure.

Typical Changes Involving the Right Coronary Artery
(See Fig. 80)

Again, when the standard leads 2 and 3 are recorded during the injection of contrast material into the right coronary artery, one notices a decrease in the heart rate as well as a decrease in the amplitude of the Q wave and of the QRS complex. More characteristically, however, the T wave in leads 2 and 3 demonstrates a decrease in amplitude or an inversion.[1,2] The Q-T interval is also prolonged.

With selective right coronary arteriography, the frontal plane mean QRS vector shifts in a clockwise manner to the right and the T wave vector shifts in a counterclockwise manner to the left.[3]

Changes Involving Abnormal Coronary Arteries

Injection of contrast into an occluded vessel is often associated with diminished or absent electrocardiographic responses. Many feel that the more normal a coronary artery, the greater the electrocardiographic changes. Biphasic electrocardiographic responses are also seen when collateral flow takes place from one coronary artery to the other. In such cases, the characteristic QRS, ST, and T wave changes for the injected coronary artery are initially elicited but subsequently the electrocardiographic changes are characteristic for the injection of the contralateral vessel. For instance, if the right coronary artery is occluded proximally and distal flow to the right coronary artery distribution is provided by collaterals from the left coronary artery, an injection of the left coronary artery may produce first an elevation of the T wave with subsequent decrease and inversion of that T wave (see Fig. 81). This means that initially the electrocardiographic changes are those of the left coronary arteriogram, whereas in the late phase the contrast is shunted to the right where it produces characteristic changes for a right coronary arteriogram.

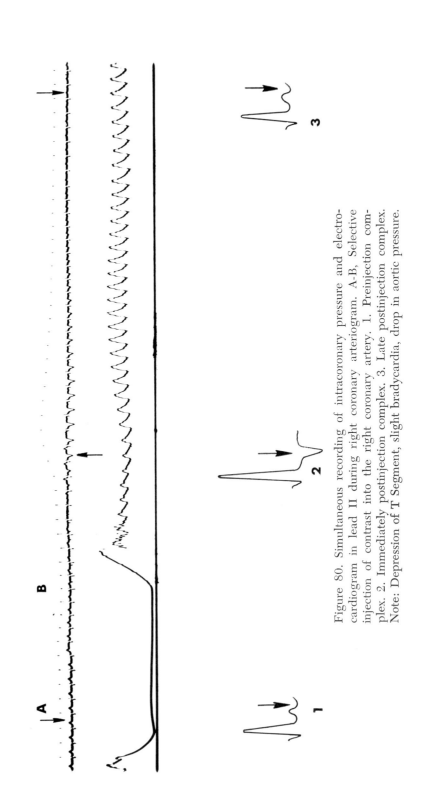

Figure 80. Simultaneous recording of intracoronary pressure and electrocardiogram in lead II during right coronary arteriogram. A-B, Selective injection of contrast into the right coronary artery. 1. Preinjection complex. 2. Immediately postinjection complex. 3. Late postinjection complex. Note: Depression of T Segment, slight bradycardia, drop in aortic pressure.

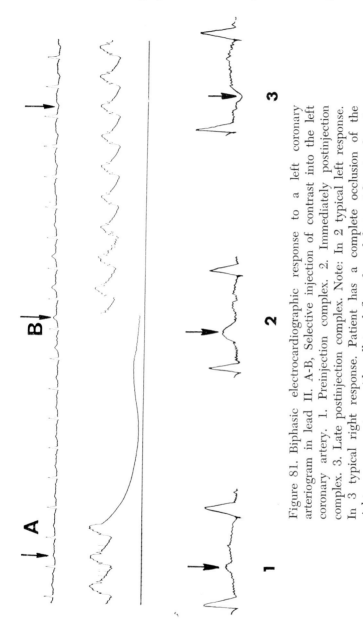

Figure 81. Biphasic electrocardiographic response to a left coronary arteriogram in lead II. A-B, Selective injection of contrast into the left coronary artery. 1. Preinjection complex. 2. Immediately postinjection complex. 3. Late postinjection complex. Note: In 2 typical left response. In 3 typical right response. Patient has a complete occlusion of the right coronary artery with collateral flow from left to right via the circumflex coronary artery.

Conduction Changes

The most common change in rhythm is the slowing of the sinus node pacemaker. The greatest slowing seems to occur after the injection of the right coronary artery. If the right coronary artery is occluded, however, greater slowing occurs during the injection of the left. Ectopic ventricular beats are rarely seen.

The occurrence of ventricular fibrillation and ventricular tachycardia is discussed in the chapter dealing with complications.

Conclusions

The electrocardiographic changes which occur during the selective injection of contrast material into coronary arteries are rather specific and helpful. During a blind injection of contrast into the coronary artery when the patient is placed over a rapid changer, electrocardiographic changes, when present, indicate that an adequate injection was administered. It is likely that the degree of electrocardiographic response is related to both the amount of myocardium perfused and also to the concentration and amount of contrast material administered. This would explain why individuals with normal coronary arteries have a greater response to the contrast material than those with occluded vessels. Curiously, it is our impression that the response to the first injection is greater than to subsequent injections. This seems also to have been the experience of Guzman and West[4] in dogs but is not supported by MacAlpin[2] *et al.*

HEMODYNAMIC CHANGES

The injection of contrast material into the coronary arteries has a toxic effect upon the myocardium.[5] This response can be quantitated by recording left ventricular pressures during the selective coronary arteriogram. A typical recording is shown in Figure 82. ECG and pressure changes occur within one or two beats after the start of the injection. Bradycardia and drop in

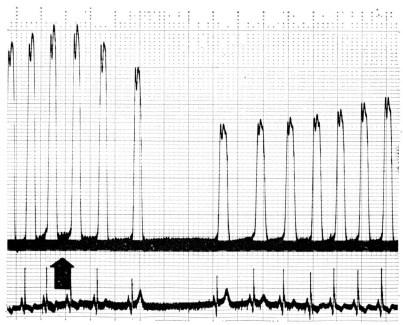

Figure 82. Marked but typical response of ECG in lead 2 and left ventricular pressure to an injection of 8 cc of 60% meglumine diatrizoate into the left coronary. Arrow indicates the beginning of injection.

peak systolic pressure are constant findings. These changes gradually return to normal in the healthy patient within ten to thirty seconds. Elevation of the end diastolic pressure is also noted but this is generally of longer duration. If the myocardium, however, is damaged, return to a preinjection status will be delayed.[6] The pressure and ECG response to the injection of a sodium salt of diatrizoate is always more marked than the meglumine salt (see Fig. 83). It should be realized that the Valsalva maneuver also produces a transient drop in systolic pressure which will in turn produce an additive effect to that of the contrast medium. Such a Valsalva maneuver is often involuntarily performed by the patient who is asked to "take in a deep breath and hold it."

The marked hyperosmolarity of the contrast material is thought to be responsible for an increase in cardiac output and a decrease of the systemic vascular resistance during the intracoronary in-

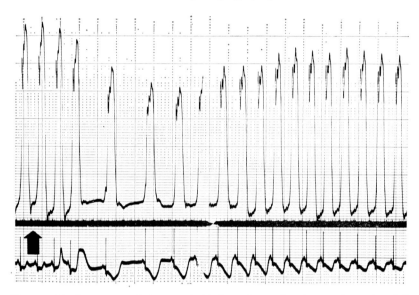

Figure 83. Injection of 8 cc of 50% sodium diatrizoate into the left coronary artery. Note the initial rise of the ST segment and the subsequent abnormal electrocardiographic response. Figures 82 and 83 were given to us by Dr. Robert Jeffery.

jection of any contrast agent. Kloster *et al.*,[7] have shown recently, that coronary arteriography increases significantly myocardial blood flow. The percentage change was 35.7% at 3 minutes after the injection, remained 32.1% after 5 minutes and returned to preinjection flows at 7 minutes. The authors interpret this change as a defense mechanism against the ischemia caused by the contrast agent.

REFERENCES

1. Coskey, R.L. and Magidson, O.: Electrocardiographic response to selective coronary arteriography. *Brit. Heart J.*, 29:512–19, 1967.
2. MacAlpin, R.N., Weidner, W.A., Kattus, A.A. Jr., and Hanafee, W.N.: Electrocardiographic changes during selective coronary cineangiography. *Circulation*, 34:627–37, 1966.
3. Smith, R.F., Harthorne, W., Sanders, C.A.: Vectorcardiographic changes during intracoronary injections. *Circulation*, 36:63–75, 1967.
4. Guzman, S.V. and West, J.W.: Cardiac effects of intracoronary arterial

injections of various roentgenographic contrast media. *Am. Heart J.*, 58:597, 1959.

5. Gensini, G.G. and DiGiorgi, S.: Myocardial toxicity of contrast agents used in angiography. *Am. J. Roentgen.*, 82:24–34, 1964.

6. Gensini, G.G., Dubiel, J., Huntington, P.P., and Kelly, A.E.: Left ventricular end-diastolic pressure before and after coronary arteriography. The value of coronary arteriography as a stress test. *Am. J. Cardiol.*, 27:453–59, 1971.

7. Kloster, F.E., Friesen, G.W., Green, S.G., and Judkins, M.P.: Effects of coronary arteriography on myocardial blood flow. *Circulation*, 46:438–444, 1972.

CHAPTER VIII

CORONARY ATHEROSCLEROSIS, COLLATERAL CIRCULATION AND THEIR EFFECT ON THE LEFT VENTRICULOGRAM

CORONARY ATHEROSCLEROSIS

The vast preponderence of coronary artery disease is due to atherosclerosis. Congenital coronary artery anomalies are ocassionally encountered; these have been discussed earlier. Other acquired diseases which can affect the coronary arteries[1] include syphilitic aortitis, medial cystic necrosis, subacute bacterial endocarditis, arteritis due to various collagen diseases, thrombotic thrombocytopenic purpura, amyloid and fibromuscular hyperplasia. All these lesions are extremely rare in comparison with atherosclerosis and thus when we speak of "coronary artery disease" patients, we are referring primarily to those with atherosclerotic processes.

Types of Atherosclerotic Disease

The most important type of atherosclerotic lesion is the *stenosing or occlusive lesion*. Atherosclerotic stenosis of a coronary artery is generally considered significant when a 50 per cent narrowing can be demonstrated at angiography.[2] Angiographers and surgeons have generally accepted this as the point where symptoms may begin to occur and where consideration of surgical therapy should be undertaken.

Narrowing can be chronic, acute, or sub-acute in nature. Chronic narrowing is caused by atherosclerotic deposits or plaques.* This is probably the most common form of atherosclerotic narrowing seen on coronary angiograms. Acute ob-

---

* These plaques can be concentric but more often are excentric.

struction is caused by sudden thrombosis or emboli. Angiographic demonstration of acute thrombosis of a major coronary artery is rare, since these patients either die suddenly or are considered too acutely ill to undergo angiographic study. An example of acute thrombosis of the right coronary artery is seen in Figure 84. Subacute or combined lesions consist of chronic atherosclerotic deposits which cause slowing and turbulence of blood flow, leading ultimately to acute thrombosis. Hemorrhage into a preexisting atherosclerotic plaque may produce a similar result.

One very important fact which must be kept in mind by the angiographer in his evaluation of narrowed coronary arteries is that thromboses of these vessels are capable of recanalizing. Although this point is often overlooked or ignored, it has been unequivocally proven by several investigators.[3-5] It is virtually impossible to differentiate angiographically between a recanalized thrombus and localized atherosclerotic stenosis.

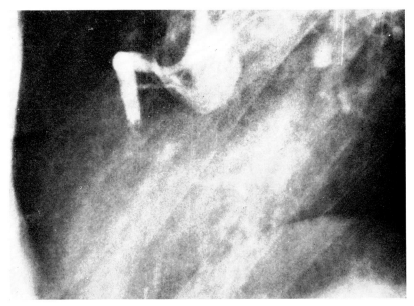

Figure 84. Acute thrombosis shortly beyond the origin of the right coronary artery, as seen on a lateral projection.

What appears to be a severe localized narrowing may represent a chronically diseased artery which has not yet occluded, or one which has undergone sub-acute or even acute thrombosis and then recanalized. Figure 85 is a graphic illustration of this dilemma. An initial coronary arteriogram showed total occlusion of the right coronary artery. Two years later, a repeat study showed this vessel to be patent except for a rather typical-looking "localized stenosis." At autopsy a short time later, this was found to be a recanalized thrombus. The inability to reliably differentiate between these two entities may explain some of the clinical paradoxes inherent in the study of coronary artery disease. This point will be discussed later in this chapter.

2. *Irregular dilatation or ectasia* is another form of coronary atherosclerosis. Here too, slowing of flow and turbulence are

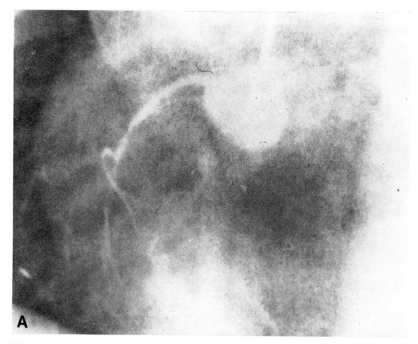

Figure 85. A, LAO view of a cine right coronary arteriogram showing total occlusion of the vessel. B, Two years later a repeat study shows localized narrowing (white arrow) where the previously occluding thrombus has undergone recanalization. C, Histologic section through the recanalized segment.   ≫

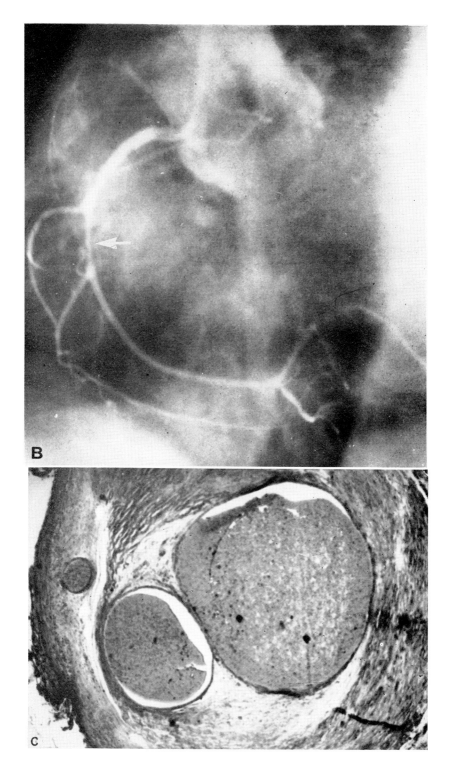

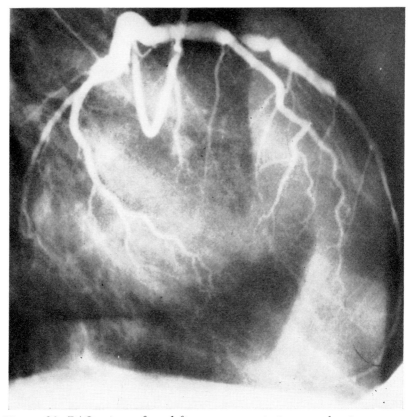

Figure 86. RAO view of a left coronary arteriogram showing severe atherosclerotic ectasia of the proximal portion of the anterior descending artery.

produced. Occasionally this lesion may progress to actual aneurysm formation. Figure 86 is an example of severe irregular dilatation of the proximal portion of an anterior descending artery.

3. *Ulceration of plaques* is a relatively rare occurrence but can be dangerous by predisposing to dislodgement with embolization, hemorrhage into the plaque itself, or dissection of the wall of the artery.

Location of Atherosclerotic Disease

In general, most patients with coronary artery disease have involvement of more than one vessel. Gensini and Buonnano[5] found that 88 per cent had angiographically demonstrable atherosclerosis in at least two major coronary arteries. The right and anterior descending coronaries are the more frequently affected, the circumflex artery to a lesser extent. Figure 87 is an example of multiple vessel involvement. There is total occlusion of both the circumflex and anterior descending arteries with flow through a patent diagonal artery.

The majority of stenosing lesions, but by no means all, are found within the proximal half of the involved artery. It is not uncommon to find severe disease in this proximal portion with the distal segment having a remarkably normal appearance. Figures 88 and 89 exemplify this.

An interesting example of localized and usually proximal coronary atherosclerosis is the "variant" form of angina pectoris described by Prinzmetal *et al.*[6] This syndrome is characterized by angina attacks which occur at rest or during light activity and which are accompanied by transient ST segment elevation. This electrocardiographic abnormality disappears when the chest pain ceases or is relieved by nitroglycerin. These patients generally have a single lesion of one of the major coronary arteries, the location of which can be predicted by the pattern of ST segment elevation among the various EKG leads. A coronary arteriogram of a patient with variant angina pectoris is shown in Figure 89.

Special mention should be made of narrowing of the left main coronary artery before its bifurcation into the anterior descending and circumflex branches. This is the most ominous of all coronary stenoses, since occlusion in this area is generally fatal. The discovery of such a lesion (Fig. 90) is often considered an indication for emergency bypass surgery.

In another and less frequent type of disease pattern, the obstructing lesion is located in the distal segment of the artery. Figure 91 shows occlusion of the right coronary artery just beyond the origin of the posterior descending branch. Lesions of the distally located left posterolateral branches of dominant right coronary arteries may prove especially troublesome to the inexperienced angiographer. These branches, which supply blood to the posterior diaphragmatic aspect of the left ventricle,

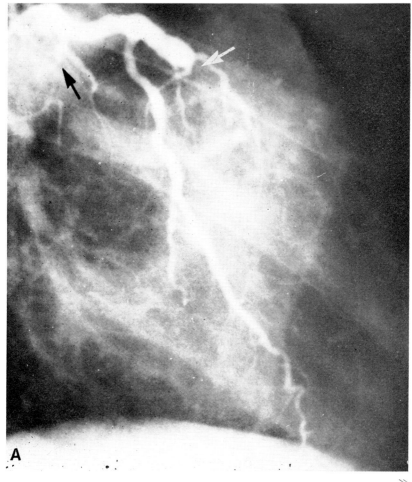

≫

are very variable in number and course and may not be missed if they are occluded at their origin. Figure 92 is an illustration of such a case. At first glance the entire right coronary artery tree appears patent, but closer scrutiny reveals occlusion of the terminal left posterolateral branch.

A third type of disease pattern is severe diffuse involvement of the entire length of the vessel (see Figs. 93 and 94). As Eckstein has pointed out,[7] resistance to flow increases as the length of the narrowed segment increases. Thus patients in this category may have disabling symptoms even though there are no localized stenoses of severe degree.

Finally, mention should be made of the puzzling group of patients who have normal coronary arteriograms in spite of strong electrocardiographic, metabolic, or clinical evidence of myocardial ischemia. These individuals have been studied by a number of investigators[1,8] but the etiology of their disease re-

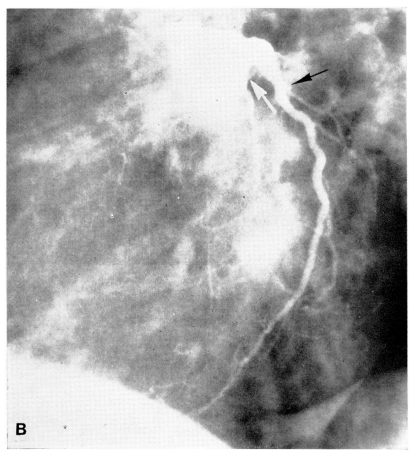

Figure 87. A, RAO and B, LAO view of a left coronary arteriogram. The black arrow points to a total occlusion of the circumflex artery and a white arrow to a total occlusion of the anterior descending artery. A large diagonal branch of the anterior descending artery supplies blood to the anterolateral wall of the left ventricle.

mains an enigma. Some of them probably have obstructive disease of coronary artery branches which are too small to be visualized at arteriography.

COLLATERAL CIRCULATION

In the presence of severe obstructing coronary atherosclerosis some degree of collateral circulation is generally found. Thorough knowledge of these collateral pathways is very helpful in differentiating between normal and pathologic circula-

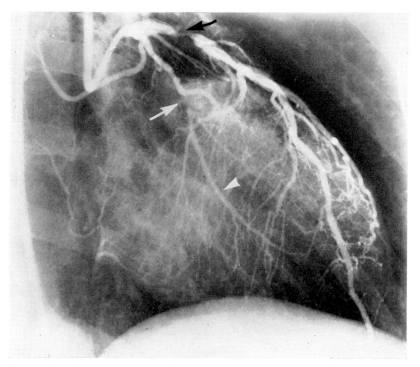

Figure 88. RAO view of a left coronary arteriogram. There is severe stenosis of the proximal portion of the anterior descending artery (black arrow). Beyond this localized lesion the vessel is normally patent. The white arrow points to a complete obstruction of the circumflex artery. The obtuse marginal branch of the circumflex artery (white arrowhead) fills retrograde via collaterals coming primarily from the diagnoal branches of the anterior descending artery.

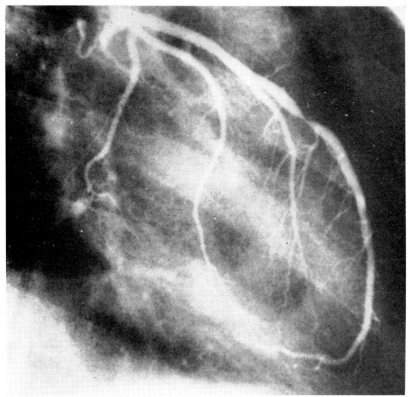

Figure 89. RAO view of a left coronary arteriogram showing a severe localized stenosis 7 cm beyond the origin of the anterior descending artery. Distally, this vessel is normally patent. Aside from the anterior descending artery, the patient's coronary circulation was entirely normal. Clinically this thirty-year-old male had Prinzmetal's variant angina pectoris and this represents the classical angiographic finding of the syndrome.

tion, evaluating the patient's symptomatology and cardiac function, and considering him as a possible surgical candidate. Often the problem of demonstrating an obstruction in a small coronary artery branch is obviated by the observation of collateral flow into the area from another nearby branch. This particular aspect of coronary angiography may indeed prove to be a much greater challenge to the angiographer than the mere identification of atherosclerotic lesions in large vessels. Accordingly we will discuss it at some length.

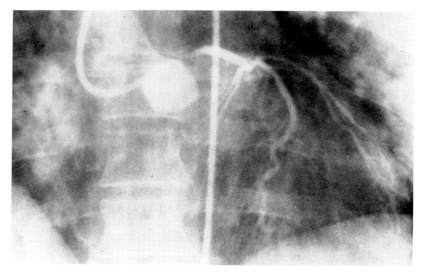

Figure 90. Stenosis of the origin of the left coronary artery. This study was obtained shortly after the administration of nitroglycerin and the lesion was therefore thought to be organic, rather than the result of spasm induced by the catheter tip.

The basis for the formation of coronary collaterals is the presence of preexisting coronary arterial anastomoses which have been shown by Baroldi and Scommazoni[4] and others to be present in the normal heart. They describe both "homocoronary" anastomoses connecting various branches of the same coronary artery and "intercoronary" anastomoses connecting branches of the three different major coronary arteries. These anastomotic vessels range in diameter up to 350 micra and in length up to 3 cm. Histologically these vessels seem to be quite different from normal coronary arteries and arterioles. They possess only an endothelial lining, and occasionally very thin medial and adventitial layers. Thus, they resemble capillaries histologically, even though they are of arteriolar or arterial size. These interconnecting anastomoses serve little function in healthy hearts and cannot be demonstrated angiographically because there is very little flow within them.[9] However, with the progressive development of coronary atherosclerosis, they serve as the precursors of the collateral circulation. It is of historical interest

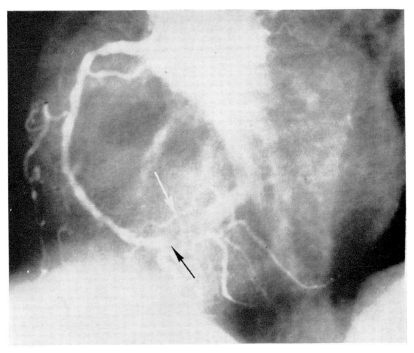

Figure 91. LAO view of a preponderant right coronary artery showing complete occlusion (black arrow) just beyond the origin of the posterior descending artery. A collateral branch which bridges the obstruction is clearly visible (white arrow).

to note that until relatively recently, normal coronary arteries were considered end-arteries without interconnecting anastomoses.[10]

Generally two stimuli are thought to cause the development of coronary collaterals.[4,11] The first is metabolic, based upon myocardial anoxia, and is poorly understood. The second is hydrodynamic, based upon the pressure relationships in different portions of the coronary tree. With the development of an obstructing lesion in a major coronary artery, the perfusion pressure drops in the distal segment. This creates a pressure gradient between the distal segment and either the proximal segment of the same artery or a nearby unobstructed coronary artery. In this situation, active flow will begin to pass from the

high pressure to the low pressure channels through the preexisting homocoronary or intercoronary anastomotic vessels.
Under the stress of increased pulsatile flow these vessels become dilated and elongated and often pursue a very tortuous
course because of their thin walls.[12] Their diameters can increase to 2 mm (occasionally even larger) and by this time

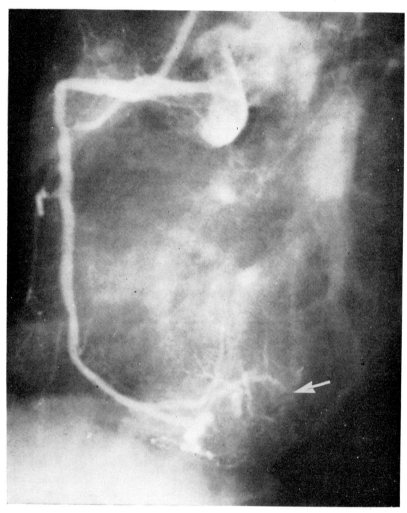

Figure 92. LAO view of a preponderant right coronary artery. Although
the posterior descending artery is patent, there is complete obstruction
of an important left posterolateral branch (white arrow).

they can be easily recognized as collaterals on the coronary arteriogram. If one examines the heart of such patients, he will find numerous congested vessels which histologically resemble capillaries but which are of arteriolar or arterial size.

Gensini and Da Costa have pointed out[9] that in order for collateral circulation to develop, severe coronary artery narrowing must be present with at least 90 per cent reduction in diameter (bearing in mind that a 90% reduction in diameter constitutes a 99% reduction in cross-sectional area). In the presence of less severe stenosis, it is extremely unlikely that collateral flow can be angiographically demonstrated. In an

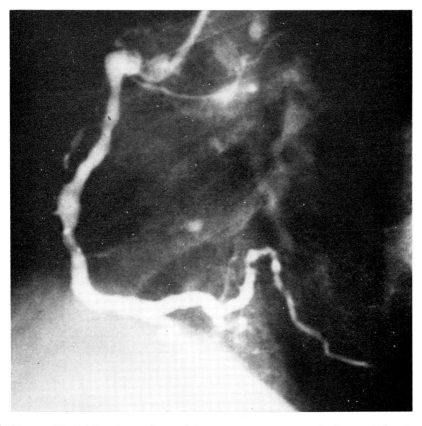

Figure 93. LAO view of a right coronary artery which is diffusely diseased along its entire length.

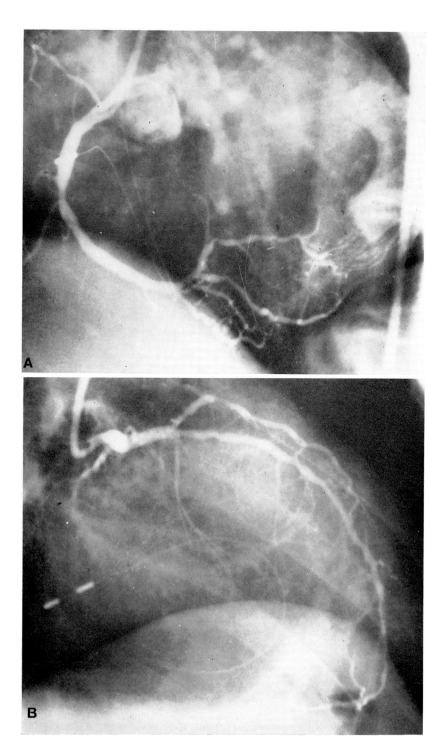

earlier study, Gensini and Buonanno[5] found that about 75 per
cent of the completely occluded arteries show some distal
opacification via collaterals. Abrams and Adams,[2] however, state
that complete occlusion is almost always accompanied by at
least some collateralization to supply the segment distal to the
block. This has also been the experience of the present authors.
The relatively rare occurrence of total lack of distal flow is invariably accompanied by severe scarring or aneurysm formation of the affected portion of the ventricle.

The development of collateral circulation may be considered
part of a process of revascularization of an area of ischemic
myocardium. Another type of revascularization previously referred to which does not truly fall into the category of collateral
circulation is recanalization of an obstructing thrombus.

Thus, a localized occlusion of any major coronary artery may
reopen by recanalization or be bypassed by various collateral
pathways.

The remainder of this section will discuss true collateral circulation of the homocoronary and intercoronary types when one
or another of the major arteries is obstructed. These pathways
have been arranged roughly in order of decreasing frequency
in our experience.

Collateral Pathways in Obstruction of a Dominant
Right Coronary Artery (Figs. 105–106 drawings A to L)

A. *Direct Bridging Collaterals*

A phenomenon which angiographically is closely related to recanalization but different pathophysiologically is the development of a network of tiny bridging vessels which pass around

≪

Figure 94. A, LAO view of a right coronary artery showing a severe
stenosis within its midportion and severe diffuse atherosclerotic disease of
all its branches along the diaphragmatic surface. B, RAO view of the left
coronary artery in the same patient. There is extensive atherosclerosis
of the entire anterior descending artery and its diagonal branch. The
circumflex artery is small due to preponderance of the right coronary
artery but is also diffusely diseased.

the occluded segment. James[12] has suggested that these may not represent true homocoronary collaterals but rather enlarged vasa vasorum in the wall of the coronary artery. This point has not been definitely established. Sometimes instead of a network, a single bridging homocoronary anastomosis is seen. Such a vessel may be several centimeters in length and pass from prestenotic to poststenotic segments of the obstructed coronary artery. Figure 105A (which is actually a diagramatic representation of Fig. 91) shows a homocoronary collateral bridging an obstructed segment of the distal right coronary artery. This type of pathway can be present in any of the three major coronary artery distributions.

B.   Distal Circumflex to Distal Right Coronary Artery

This common pathway is illustrated in Figure 105B and Figure 95. Right coronary obstruction is often accompanied by the presence of collateral branches from the distal circumflex artery to the distal left atrioventricular extension of the right coronary artery. The latter fills in a retrograde direction. The frequency of this pathway is due to the fact that these arteries normally terminate quite closely to one another along the diaphragmatic aspect of the left atrioventricular groove.

C.   Left Atrial Circumflex to Distal Right or AV Node Artery

Where the circumflex artery is small, a branch of the nearby left atrial circumflex may anastomose either directly with the distal right coronary artery or with its AV node branch. The former arrangement is illustrated in Figure 105C. Figure 95 shows collaterals from both the circumflex and left atrial circumflex arteries filling the distal right coronary artery in a retrograde direction.

D.   Obtuse Marginal or Diagonal to Left Posterolateral Branch

Frequently the last major branch of a dominant right coronary artery before its termination along the left atrioventricular groove is a large left posterolateral artery. The latter supplies the diaphragmatic aspect of the posterior left ventricle and can receive collateral flow from either the obtuse marginal branch of the left circumflex artery or the diagonal branch of the left anterior descending artery. Figure 105D illustrates a collateral connection between the obtuse marginal and left posterolateral branches.

E. Anterior Descending to Posterior Descending Artery Through the Ventricular Septum

Both the anterior descending and posterior descending arteries supply a rich network of septal arteries. With obstruction of the right coronary artery this septal network provides a commonly utilized collateral pathway by which blood passes from the anterior descending to the posterior descending artery. Figure 105E and Figure 96 illustrate this. In the case shown in Figure 96, there was very little filling of the post-stenotic distal segment of the right main coronary artery from either side. However, the left coronary injection resulted in good filling of the posterior descending branch through septal collaterals.

F. High Acute Marginal to Low Acute Marginal Arteries

There are often two acute marginal branches of the right coronary artery. When a right main coronary obstruction develops between their origins, collateral vessels may connect them, thereby bypassing the obstruction. See Figure 105F and Figure 97.

G. Conus to Acute Marginal Artery

When only a single acute marginal artery is present and obstruction develops proximal to it, a pathway similar to the one described above may be seen. Instead of a connection between two marginal branches, there is a connection between the conus artery and the acute marginal artery. See Figure 105G.

H. Kugel's Artery

This well known but rarely demonstrated pathway was first described in 1927 by Kugel[13] who called it the arteria anastomotica auricularis magna. It is a small vessel which can originate from either the proximal right or left coronary artery, then passes down the anterior margin of the atrial septum to anastomose with the AV node artery, which in turn originates from the distal right coronary at the crux of the heart. It is thus capable of bypassing any obstruction of the proximal or midportion of a dominant right coronary artery. Figure 105H and Figure 98 show the course of this vessel.

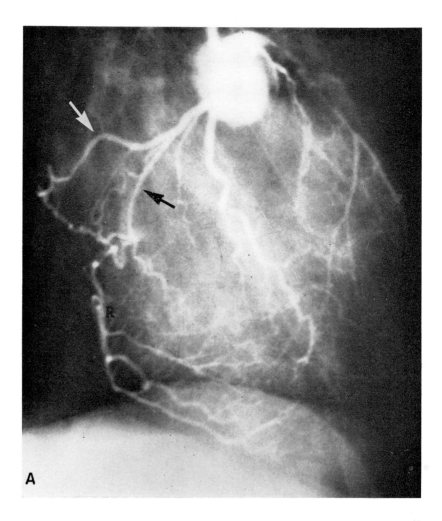

A

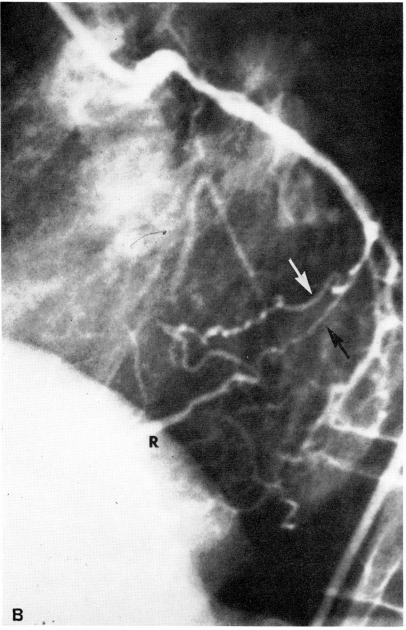

B

Figure 95. A, RAO and B, LAO views of the left coronary artery showing complete occlusion of the anterior descending artery. This patient
also had a complete occlusion of the proximal portion of his preponderant
right coronary artery. Note filling of the distal right coronary artery (R)
and its posterior descending and left posterolateral branches via collaterals
from the left circumflex (black arrows) and left atrial circumflex arteries
(white arrows).

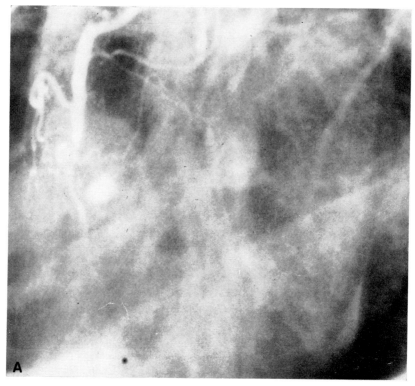

≫

I. SA Node Artery to Left Atrial to Distal Right Coronary Artery

This very rare but striking collateral pathway is shown in Figure 105I and Figure 99. In this case, right coronary obstruction was present just beyond the origin of the SA node artery. The latter gives off a large collateral branch connecting with the left atrial circumflex artery which in turn feeds the terminal portion of the right coronary artery.

J. Left Anterior Descending to Acute Marginal Artery

This is also very rare. The normal anterior descending artery may give rise to several very small branches to the anterior surface of the right ventricle. In proximal right coronary obstruction, one of them may enlarge and connect with the acute marginal artery. Blood can then pass from this right ventricular branch retrograde through the acute marginal artery to fill the distal right coronary artery, as shown in Figure 106J.

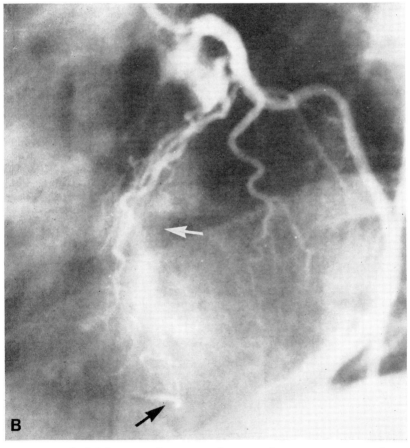

Figure 96. A, LAO view of a preponderant right coronary artery showing nearly total occlusion. B, LAO view of the left coronary arteriogram in the same patient. Collaterals are seen extending down the interventricular septum (white arrow) from the anterior descending artery to supply the posterior descending branch (black arrow) of the right coronary artery.

K. Left Anterior Descending Around the Apex to Posterior Descending Artery

Both the anterior and posterior descending arteries usually terminate near the cardiac apex, the former along the anterior interventricular groove and the latter along the posterior interventricular groove. Not infrequently, however, the posterior descending artery is short and only passes half way down the posterior interventricular groove. In these cases the anterior

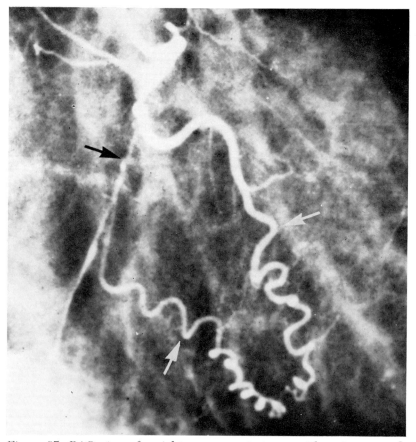

Figure 97. RAO view of a right coronary arteriogram. There is a severely narrowed segment (black arrow) which is being bypassed by collateral connections between large acute marginal branches (white arrows) on either side of it.

descending artery passes completely around the apex to terminate along the diaphragmatic aspect of the heart. This is the normal course of the artery and should not be misconstrued as a collateral. In rare instances of obstruction of the right coronary artery or posterior descending artery, a collateral pathway *will* be seen from the anterior descending artery around the apex to the distal posterior descending artery. (See Figure 106K.) Tortuosity of the anastomotic vessel and visualization of right coronary or posterior descending obstruction provide evidence that the pathway is a collateral rather than a normal channel.

L. Low Acute Marginal to Posterior Descending Artery

A final rare collateral pathway in cases of distal right coronary or proximal posterior descending obstruction is through a low acute marginal artery, as illustrated in Figure 106L. These low marginal branches often course obliquely across the diaphragmatic surface of the right ventricle towards the septum and can anastomose with the nearby distal posterior descending artery to bypass the obstruction.

Collateral Pathways in Obstruction of the Left Anterior Descending Artery (Figs. 106–107 drawings M to T)

The formation of bridging collaterals also occurs within the left anterior descending distribution.

M. Conus to Left Anterior Descending Artery

This classical collateral circle, illustrated in Figure 100 and Figure 106M, was originally described by Vieussens in 1706.[14] The conus artery originates from the proximal right coronary artery in roughly half of all human hearts and directly from the aorta in the vicinity of the right coronary ostium in the other half. When the proximal anterior descending artery is occluded, injection of the right coronary artery will often opacify it through collaterals from the conus branch. Even where the conus branch has a separate aortic orifice, there is generally enough reflux of contrast out into the right sinus of Valsalva to fill it. Sometimes a separate injection into the cusp itself must be made to locate it.

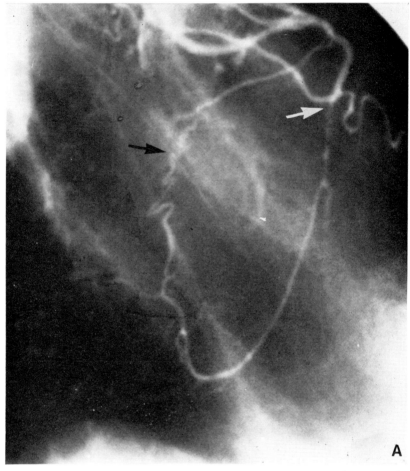

A

≫

Figure 98. (A) RAO view and (B) AP view of a preponderant right coronary artery. The white arrow points to a severe stenosis within the proximal portion of this vessel. The black arrow points to Kugel's artery which connects the pre-stenotic segment of the right coronary artery with the A-V node artery.

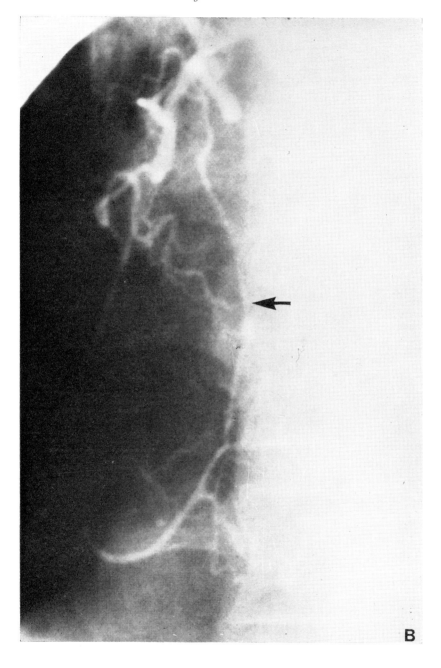

N.   *Acute Marginal to Left Anterior Descending Artery*

This is another common intercoronary collateral pathway from the right side to the left anterior descending artery and is quite similar to the circle of Vieussens. Figure 101 and Figure 106N illustrate it.

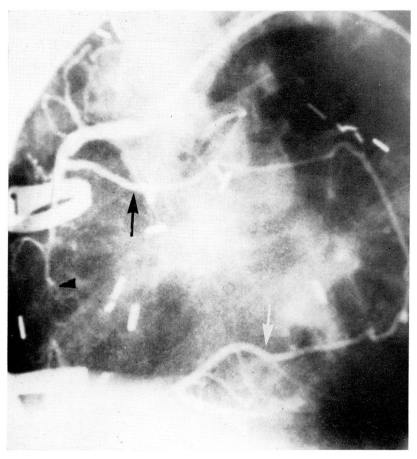

Figure 99. LAO view of a right coronary arteriogram in a patient who had undergone a previous Vineberg operation. The right coronary artery is totally occluded (black arrowhead). A long collateral connection can be seen between the S-A node artery (black arrow) and the distal right coronary (white arrow) by way of the left atrial circumflex artery.

O. Proximal Septal to Distal Septal Branches

The first interventricular septal branch of the left anterior descending artery is often a large one and obstructions often occur just beyond its take-off. In this situation blood may flow down the proximal septal branch through a collateral network in the septum itself and then retrograde back up more distal septal branches to fill the post-obstructive segment of the left anterior descending artery. This is shown in Figure 102 and Figure 106O.

P. Obtuse Marginal to Diagonal Branch

The left anterior descending artery may have one or more diagonal branches passing over the lateral wall of the left ventricle. The obtuse marginal branch of the circumflex artery also supplies the lateral wall of the left ventricle. When the terminal ramifications of the diagonal and marginal branches are close together, a proximal anterior descending block can be circumvented by collateral flow from the marginal to the diagonal branch. Flow then passes back to the anterior descending artery itself. See Figure 103 and Figure 106P.

Q. Obstuse Marginal to Left Anterior Descending Artery

This pathway is illustrated by Figure 106Q. It is similar to the pathway described in the previous paragraph but less frequently encountered. Here the collateral flow is from the marginal branch directly to the distal anterior descending artery, a somewhat longer route.

R. Posterior Descending Around the Apex to the Left Anterior Descending Artery

This is the converse of the pathway shown in Figure 106K and, like it, is seen infrequently. Figure 100 and Figure 106R illustrate this pattern. Figure 100 shows an occluded anterior descending artery opacifying through both the conus and posterior descending arteries, emphasizing the point that two or even more separate collateral pathways can be utilized at the same time.

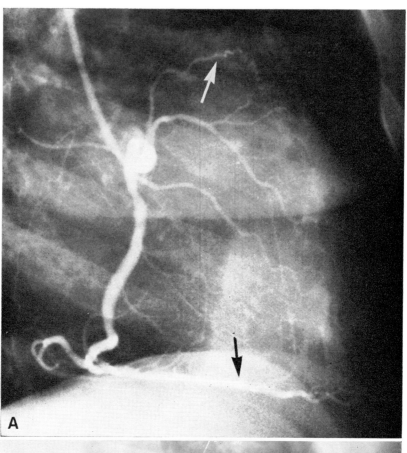

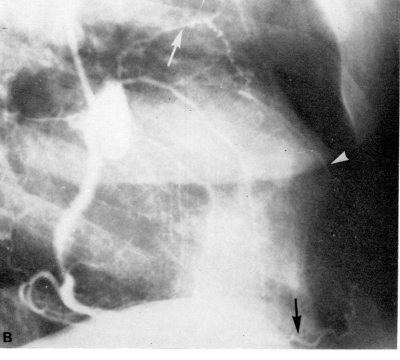

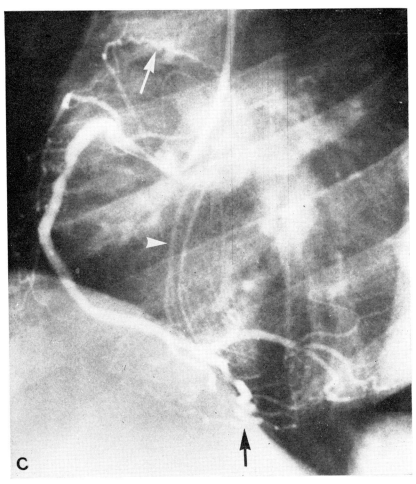

Figure 100. A and B, Early and late phase RAO view of the right coronary artery. C, LAO view of the right coronary artery. This patient had total occlusion of the left anterior descending artery. The distal anterior descending (white arrowhead) is seen to fill on this injection via collaterals from the conus artery (white arrow) and the distal end of the posterior descending artery (black arrow).

≪

S. *Posterior Descending to Anterior Descending Arteries Through to the Ventricular Septum*

This is the converse of the pathway shown in Figure 105E but is seen only very rarely. See Figure 107S.

T. *Diagonal Septal Branches to Anterior Descending Septal Branches*

Occasionally the anterior descending artery has a large diag-

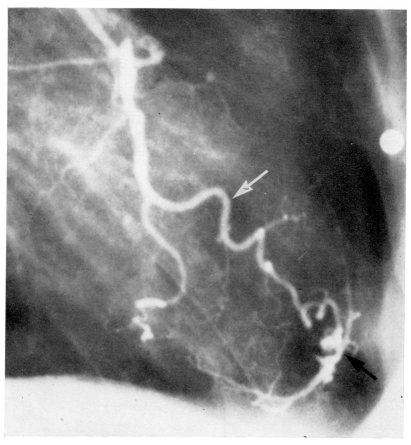

Figure 101. RAO view of the right coronary arteriogram in a patient with obstruction of the left anterior descending artery. A large acute marginal branch (white arrow) supplies collateral flow to the distal anterior descending artery (black arrow).

onal branch which closely parallels it just to the left of the interventricular groove. Because of its proximity to the interventricular septum, this diagonal artery may have a number of septal branches. In fact its course and septal ramifications may be so similar to those of the left anterior descending artery itself that occlusion of the latter could easily be overlooked. The septal branches of the diagonal artery may in this situation ana-

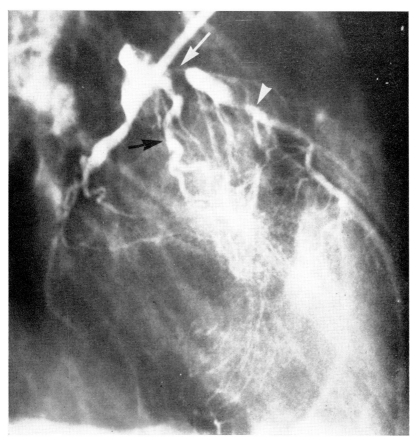

Figure 102. RAO view of the left coronary artery in a patient with obstruction of the left anterior descending artery (white arrow) just beyond the first septal branch (black arrow). Blood passes down this first septal branch, through a rich collateral network in the septum itself and then back up the more distal septal branches to the distal anterior descending artery (white arrowhead).

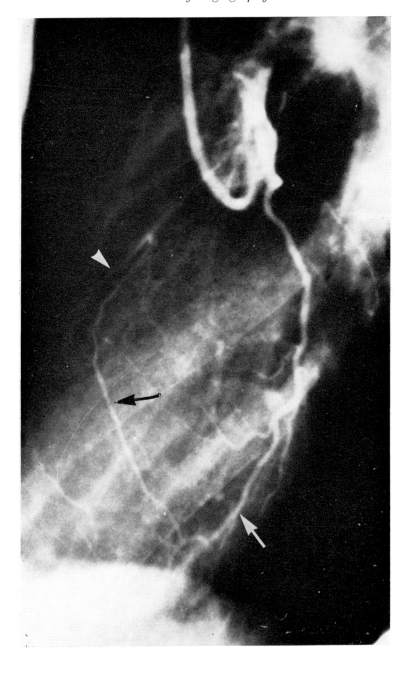

stomose with the septal branches of the anterior descending artery, thereby filling its distal segment. This pathway is illustrated in Figure 107T.

Collateral Pathways in Obstruction
of the Left Circumflex Artery (Fig. 107 drawings U to Y)

Bridging collaterals can form within the left circumflex distribution as is the case with the other two major coronary arteries. This has been discussed above.

U. *Diagonal to Obtuse Marginal Artery*

The vast majority of human subjects have preponderant right coronary arteries and in these cases the circumflex artery is small. Often it fails to extend all the way around the obtuse margin. Regardless of the size of the circumflex artery however, it usually gives off at least one large and important obtuse marginal branch which supplies the myocardium along the lateral wall of the left ventricle. Beyond the origin of the marginal branch, the circumflex itself may be a tiny and unimportant vessel. When the proximal portion of the circumflex artery is obstructed, this large obtuse marginal branch frequently derives collateral supply from the nearby diagonal branches of the left anterior descending artery. This is illustrated by Figure 88 and Figure 107U.

V. *Left Posterolateral to Obtuse Marginal Branch*

The terminal left posterolateral branches of preponderant right coronary arteries supply a variable amount of the inferior and lateral surfaces of the left ventricle. These branches may be

≪

Figure 103. Lateral view of a left coronary arteriogram in a patient with severe disease of the proximal anterior descending artery. There is collateral flow from the obtuse marginal artery (white arrow) to the diagonal branch (black arrow) of the anterior descending artery. This pathway provides a small amount of flow to the distal anterior descending artery (white arrowhead). (This case was kindly loaned to us by Dr. Robert Jeffrey of Mary Hitchcock Memorial Hospital, Hanover, New Hampshire.)

closely associated with the obtuse marginal branch and supply collateral flow to it (Figure 107V) when the circumflex artery is obstructed. This is the converse of the pathway described in Figure 105D.

W. *Distal Right to Distal Circumflex Artery*

Preponderant right coronary arteries terminate along the left atrioventricular groove near the terminal branches of the circumflex artery. When the latter is obstructed, collateral vessels supplying it in retrograde fashion from the distal right coronary artery may be seen, as shown in Figure 107W. This pathway is the converse of the one described in Figure 105B but occurs with much less frequency.

X. *High Obtuse Marginal to Low Obtuse Marginal Branch*

If there are two or more obtuse marginal branches and the circumflex artery is obstructed between their origins, anastomotic connections between the proximal and distal marginal branches may be seen circumventing it. See Figure 107X. This is analogous to the pathway described in Figure 105F.

Y. *Left Atrial Circumflex to Distal Circumflex Artery*

The left atrial circumflex artery often arises from the proximal portion of the left circumflex artery. In obstruction of the left circumflex artery, the left atrial circumflex may supply collateral flow to its distal segment through a branch running parallel to but behind the atrioventricular groove. This is shown in Figure 107Y.

Significance of Coronary Collateral Circulation

Although the anatomic features of the coronary collateral circulation have been relatively easy to document, its functional significance remains considerably more difficult to assess and numerous unsolved questions remain.[15] For instance, why is it that some patients with long-standing gradually progressive disease lack good collaterals while others have them? Why does a well-developed collateral circulation fail to protect some patients against angina, myocardial infarction, or sudden death? Should asymptomatic coronary artery disease patients with good collateral circulation be treated surgically or medically? The solutions to these and many other problems await further investigation.

In our opinion the major protective function of the collateral circulation is to prevent destruction of myocardium. Where severe coronary artery obstruction is present, some form of revascularization must occur to maintain viability of the affected muscle. This revascularization can be in the form of recanalization of a thrombus, bridging of the lesion by enlarged vasa vasorum or the presence of true collateral anastomoses—it makes relatively little difference so long as sufficient flow to the affected area continues. If there is complete lack of blood supply by any route, severe myocardial scarring occurs almost invariably (see Fig. 104). Gensini and Buonanno[5] found that 16 per cent of their patients with complete occlusion of one or more major coronary arteries had normal resting electrocardiograms. It is very likely that in many of these cases, the normal electrocardiogram was due to the presence of good collateral circulation.

LEFT VENTRICULOGRAPHY

Cine ventriculography should be carried out with every coronary arteriogram to assess left ventricular function. While a large number of physiological tests have been devised to evaluate performance of the ventricle as a whole, it is only through ventriculography that localized contractility disorders can be detected. Since coronary artery disease often affects one portion of the left ventricular myocardium more than others, the importance of ventriculography becomes obvious.

Cine ventriculography should always be performed with the patient lying in the right anterior oblique position. Of late, we have also begun performing left anterior oblique ventriculography to exclude dysfunction of the septum or lateral wall of the ventricle. Our ventriculograms are done after the completion of coronary angiography, although some prefer the reverse

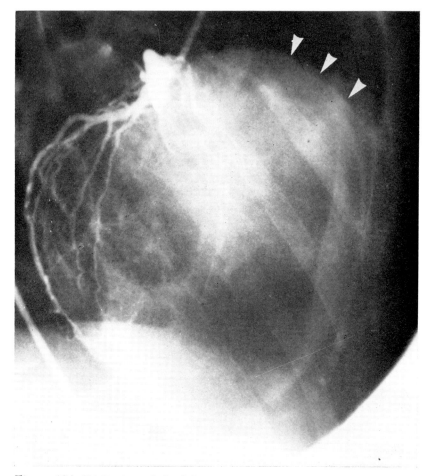

Figure 104. RAO view of the left coronary artery showing total occlusion of the anterior descending artery at its origin. There was no collateral circulation to the distal portion of this vessel from any source. The arrowheads outline the soft tissue shadow of the resultant large ventricular aneurysm of the anterior wall.

>>

Figures 105, 106, and 107 The small arrows point to obstructions of a coronary artery. RC = right coronary artery. PD = posterior descending artery. LPL = left posterolateral artery. LAD = left anterior descending artery. C = left circumflex artery. OM = obtuse marginal artery. AM = acute marginal artery. D = diagonal branch of the left anterior descending artery.

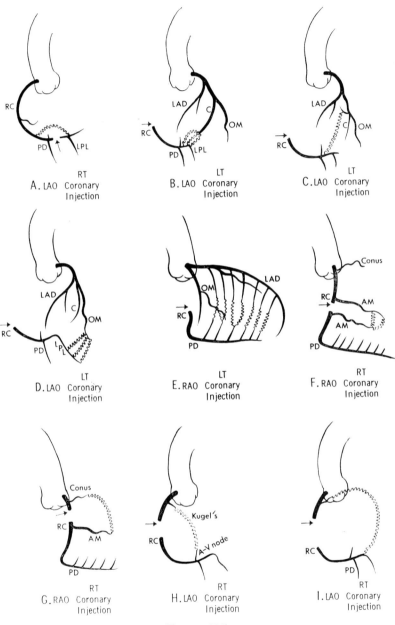

RT
A. LAO Coronary
Injection

LT
B. LAO Coronary
Injection

LT
C. LAO Coronary
Injection

LT
D. LAO Coronary
Injection

LT
E. RAO Coronary
Injection

RT
F. RAO Coronary
Injection

RT
G. RAO Coronary
Injection

RT
H. LAO Coronary
Injection

RT
I. LAO Coronary
Injection

Figure 105

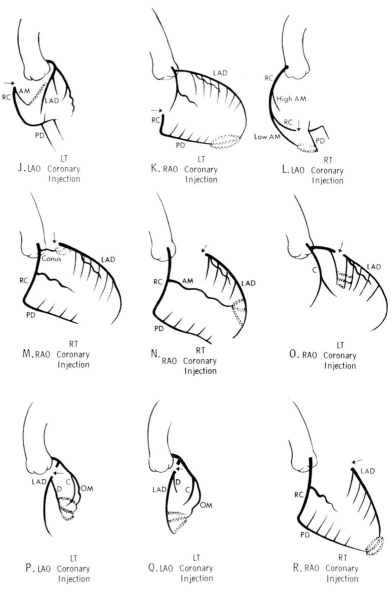

J. LT LAO Coronary Injection

K. LT RAO Coronary Injection

L. RT LAO Coronary Injection

M. RT RAO Coronary Injection

N. RT RAO Coronary Injection

O. LT RAO Coronary Injection

P. LT LAO Coronary Injection

Q. LT LAO Coronary Injection

R. RT RAO Coronary Injection

Figure 106

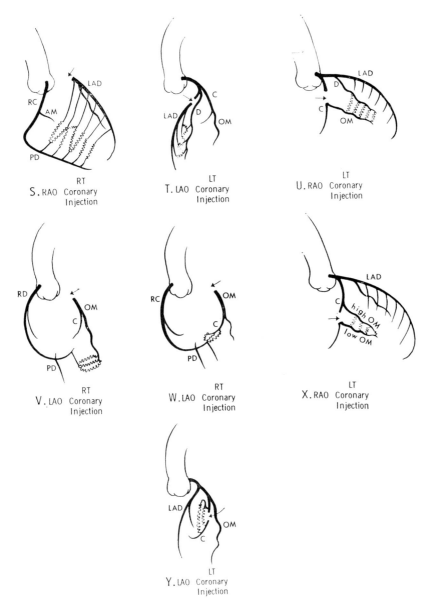

S. RAO Coronary Injection RT

T. LAO Coronary Injection LT

U. RAO Coronary Injection LT

V. LAO Coronary Injection RT

W. LAO Coronary Injection RT

X. RAO Coronary Injection LT

Y. LAO Coronary Injection LT

Figure 107

order. A "pig-tail" catheter is used for this portion of the study. This catheter configuration results in considerably less recoil during high pressure injections than occurs with straight, open-end catheters. There is also a much smaller chance of subendocardial dissection of the catheter tip during the high pressure injection. Straight, open-end catheters with side holes are used in our laboratory for ventriculography only when aortic stenosis is present, which may preclude passage of a pig-tail catheter through the valve into the left ventricle.

The catheter is generally positioned near the apex of the ventricle and a test injection of contrast material is made to see that the tip is free within the lumen. Fifty cc to sixty cc of contrast are then injected with the pressure injector. Frequently, the injection triggers a chain of premature ventricular contractions, which makes analysis of chamber function difficult. We have found that a relatively slow injection rate of 15 cc to 25 cc per second gives quite adequate ventricular filling, yet produces relatively little irritability.

In analyzing ventricular contraction, ectopic beats should be excluded from consideration. A normal systole should show an almost concentric inward motion of all points along the inner surface of the ventricle. Shortening of approximately 20 per cent occurs along the longitudinal axis and approximately 50 per cent along the transverse axis.[16] Regurgitation of contrast across the mitral valve into the left atrium is common during premature beats, but should not occur during normal systole.

The cine ventriculogram can also be used as the basis for quantitative studies of left ventricular function, such as end-diastolic volume,[17] ejection fraction and velocity of circumferential fiber shortening.

The histopathology of myocardial ischemia has been discussed by Snow *et al.*[3] They point out that in many infarcts the entire muscle mass does not become necrotic. Instead, there remains a network of surviving muscle bundles which form a living framework between the necrotic tissue. Healed infarcts may show relatively large areas of fibrous replacement alternating with areas of viable myocardium. Successive episodes of infarction of the same area will result in further destruction of the surviving muscle bundles.

Progressive ischemia without infarction will also produce myocardial fibrosis but here the replacement of muscle takes place gradually, fiber by fiber, resulting in a more homogeneous appearance which can be distinguished from that of infarction. The more severe and prolonged the ischemia, the more diffuse will be the fibrotic replacement.

In some cases, myocardium which appears to be structurally normal may lose its ability to contract properly due to lack of adequate blood supply. Herman and Gorlin[18] have postulated that in such cases ischemia may lead to abnormal conduction of the basic depolarizing impulse or cause ultrastructural changes in the mitochondria, sarcotubular system or the actin and myosin filaments. Presumably the ischemia is not severe or chronic enough to have yet produced fibrosis or infarction.

Thus an area of myocardium which appears hypokinetic or akinetic radiographically can represent an old infarct, gradually progressive ischemic fibrosis, or viable muscle which has been rendered nonfunctional by lack of adequate blood supply. It is not possible to differentiate these three conditions by ventriculography although further investigation of this matter is necessary. Postoperative ventriculography following successful direct myocardial revascularization surgery often demonstrates striking improvement in areas of previously impaired contractility.[19] Localized hypokinesia should thus by no means be considered irreversible.

Portions of the left ventricle showing dyskinetic activity (as opposed to hypokinesia or akinesia) are virtually always found to be severely scarred as a result of prior myocardial infarction. These are commonly referred to as ventricular aneurysms, a term which is appropriate since it helps differentiate them from the less severely diseased hypokinetic or akinetic areas. Ventricular aneurysms have little or no viable muscle remaining and cannot be restored to function by surgical revascularization.

The development of a hypokinetic, akinetic, or dyskinetic lesion of the left ventricular myocardium is generally the result of a complex interplay of factors, including the location and severity of coronary artery stenosis, the degree of collateral circulation present, hemoglobin-oxygen affinity, the efficiency of oxygen diffusion and utilization at the cellular level and the demands placed upon the heart itself. In many cases, localized ventricular contraction abnormalities can be satisfactorily explained by an obstructive lesion in the coronary artery supply of that particular area of myocardium. However, inconsistencies occur frequently. On the one hand we find patients with only relatively mild coronary artery stenoses exhibiting fairly abnormal ventricular contractility. In such cases, careful review of the coronary arteriogram is mandatory, to be sure that a small branch occlusion has not been overlooked. On the other hand we have seen a number of patients with severe 3-vessel coronary atherosclerosis who have entirely normal left ventricular contraction. The angiographer should expect to encounter such paradoxes fairly often and be neither surprised nor dismayed by them.

Another complication of left ventricular myocardial ischemia is the development of papillary muscle dysfunction or rupture of their chorda tendineae. This will result in mitral insufficiency and account for the systolic murmur that develops in some coronary artery disease patients.

A final rare complication is the development of an acquired interventricular septal defect. This results from severe septal infarction and necrosis. Along with the aforementioned acquired mitral insufficiency, it should be considered in differential diagnosis of systolic murmurs of sudden onset in adults with coronary artery disease.

REFERENCES

1. James, T.N.: Pathology of small coronary arteries. *Am. J. Cardiology, 20:*679–691, 1967.
2. Abrams, H.L. and Adams, D.F.: The coronary arteriogram. Structural and functional aspects. *New Engl. J. Med., 281:*1276–1285 and 1336–1342, 1969.
3. Snow, P.J.D., Jones, A.M., and Daber, K.S.: Coronary disease: A pathologic study. *Brit. Heart J., 17:*503–510, 1955.

4. Baroldi, G. and Scomazzoni, G.: Coronary circulation in the normal and the pathologic heart. Office of the Surgeon General, Department of the Army, Washington, D.C., 1967.

5. Gensini, G.G. and Buonanno, C.: Coronary arteriography. A study of 100 cases with angiographically proven coronary artery disease. *Dis. Chest*, *54*,90–99, 1968.

6. Prinzmetal, M., Ekmekci, A., Kennamer, R., Kwoczynski, J.K., Shubin, H., Toyoshima, H.: Variant form of angina pectoris. Previously undelineated syndrome. *J.A.M.A.*, *174*:1794–1800, 1960.

7. Eckstein, R.: Effect of exercise and coronary artery narrowing on coronary collateral circulation. *Circ. Res.*, 5:230–235, 1957.

8. Likoff, W., Segal, B.L., and Kasparian, H.: Paradox of normal selective coronary arteriograms in patients considered to have unmistakeable coronary artery disease. *New Engl. J. Med.*, 276:1063–1066, 1967.

9. Gensini, G.G. and DaCosta, B.C.B.: The coronary collateral circulation in living man. *Am. J. Cardiol.*, *24*:393–400, 1969.

10. Schlesinger, M.J.: An injection plus dissection study of coronary artery occlusions and anastomoses. *Am. Heart J.*, *15*:528–568, 1938.

11. Helfant, R.H., Vokonas, P.S., and Gorlin, R.: Functional importance of the human coronary collateral circulation. *New Engl. J. Med.*, *284*:1277–1281, 1971.

12. James, T.N.: Anatomy of the coronary arteries. New York, Paul B. Hoeber Inc., 1961.

13. Kugel, M.A.: Anatomical studies on the coronary arteries and their branches. I. Arteria anastomotica auricularis magna. *Am. Heart J.*, 3:260–270, 1927.

14. Vieussens, R.: *Nouvelles Decouvertes Sur Le Coeur*. Paris, 1706.

15. Sheldon, W.C.: On the significance of coronary collaterals. *Am. J. Cardiol.*, *24*:303–304, 1969.

16. Herman, M.V., Heinle, R.A., Klein, M.D., and Gorlin, R.: Localized disorders in myocardial contraction. Asynergy and its role in congestive heart failure. *New Engl. J. Med.*, 277:222–232, 1967.

17. Dodge, H.T.: Determination of left ventricular volume and mass. *Radiol. Clin. N. Am.*, 9:459–467, 1971.

18. Herman, M.V. and Gorlin, R.: Implications of left ventricular asynergy. *Am. J. Cardiol.*, 3:538–547, 1969.

19. Saltiel, J., Lesperance, J., Bourassa, M.G., Castonguay, Y., Campeau, L., and Grondin, P.: Reversibility of left ventricular dysfunction following aorto-coronary bypass vein grafts. *Am. J. Roentgen. Rad. Therap. Nucl. Med.*, *110*:739–746, 1970.

20. Bjork, L.: Angiographic demonstration of collaterals to the coronary arteries in patients with angina pectoris. *Acta Radiol Diagnosis*, 8: 305–309, 1969.

21. Likoff, W., Kasparian, H., Segal, B.L., Novack, P., and Lehman, J.S.: Clinical correlation of coronary arteriography. *Am. J. Cardiol., 16:* 159–164, 1965.
22. Paulin, S.: Interarterial coronary anastomoses in relation to arterial obstruction demonstrated in coronary arteriography. *Invest. Radiol.,* 2:147–159, 1967.
23. Schlesinger, M.J., Zoll, P.M., and Wessler, S.: The conus artery: a third coronary artery. *Am. Heart J.,* 38:823–836, 1949.
24. Zoll, P.M., Wessler, S., and Schlesinger, M.J.: Interarterial coronary anastomoses in the human heart, with particular reference to anemia and relative cardiac anoxia. *Circulation,* 4:797–815, 1951.

CHAPTER IX

THE POSTSURGICAL CORONARY ARTERIOGRAM

$\mathbf{F}$ollowing myocardial revascularization operations it is customary to perform postoperative angiograms. These consist of the opacification of the coronary arteries themselves and/or of the vessels that have been utilized to bypass an obstructed coronary artery. The first reexamination can be performed one or two weeks after surgery in the case of saphenous venous bypasses or after six to twelve months in the case of the Vineberg procedure. Subsequent yearly examinations are also recommended by some.

Coronary artery surgery can be divided into the direct and indirect revascularization techniques.

INDIRECT SURGICAL TECHNIQUES

The Vineberg procedure,[1] consisting of the implantation of the internal mammary artery into the myocardium, is one of the oldest surgical techniques used for the relief of angina. Unilateral or bilateral implantation of the internal mammary artery is performed with the hope of improving myocardial perfusion. It is commonly believed that it takes at least three to six months to develop collateral circulation. This collateral circulation presumably occurs because new blood vessels grow into the myocardium and thus bypass the diseased coronary arteries.[2] Therefore, it is customary to reexamine the patients six to twelve months after surgery.

Catheterization of the internal mammary artery was first described by Arner[3] and is a relatively easy procedure. If only one internal mammary has been anastomosed, the technique of choice is to approach the vessel from the axillary route. A catheter made of polyethylene (6–7 French) with a small pre-shaped curve can be used. When bilateral internal mammary arteries have been implanted, it is preferable to utilize the femoral approach. A right coronary catheter as described by Judkins might be adequate for both vessels. Dart *et al.*[4] have modified this catheter for transfemoral internal mammary arteriography. In patients who have severe atherosclerosis and where the innominate artery is rather tortuous, it might be impossible to pass the catheter to the origin of the internal mammary artery and the transaxillary route must therefore be used.

The injection of contrast material into the internal mammary is done by hand and the amount must not exceed 8 to 10 cc. Such an injection sometimes results in chest pain which is not due to angina, but rather to the introduction of a hypertonic solution into branches of the internal mammary artery supplying the chest wall. It is customary to perform cine angiography as well as rapid serial film radiography in both oblique projections.

Ideally, the contrast enters the myocardium and subsequently fills branches of the left coronary artery with retrograde filling to the point of stenosis (see Fig. 108). In other cases, only myocardial blushing will be observed. This, however, also represents a good surgical result (see Fig. 109). Therefore, various degrees of opacification can be seen but one must not conclude that the opacification of the internal mammary artery alone represents adequate myocardial perfusion via that vessel. At times the internal mammary artery is patent all the way to the myocardial tunnel but there is no actual communication between this tunnel and the coronary arteries or the syncytium of the myocardium. Patency of the vessel in the absence of distal runoff has been explained by the to and fro motion in the myocardial tunnel caused by cardiac contraction as well as by the mechanical defibrination.[5]

It is obvious that injections of contrast media into the internal mammary artery must be done with the same precautionary measures as when a coronary arteriogram is performed.

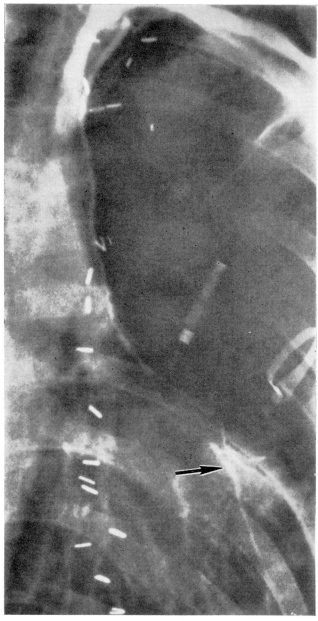

Figure 108. Left subclavian arteriogram. Note the opacification of the left internal mammary artery which has been implanted into the myocardium of the left ventricle .Note the opacification of the left anterior descending coronary artery (see arrow) via collaterals.

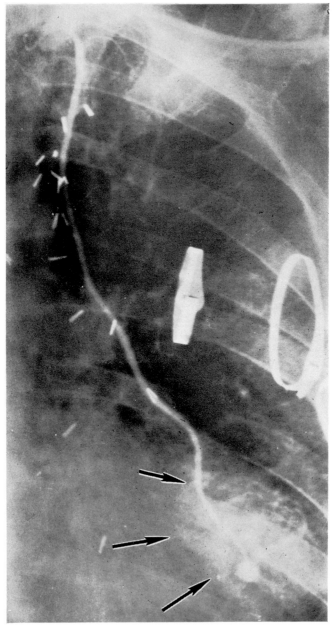

Figure 109. Post-Vineberg procedure arteriogram. The catheter is selectively placed into the left internal mammary artery. Note the myocardial blushing outlined by arrows.

In our limited experience, we have never seen ventricular fi-brillation occur during the injection of an internal mammary artery; however, one should be prepared for such a possibility. Objective criteria to indicate efficacy of the Vineberg proce-dure have been defined by Gorlin.[2] He followed one hundred patients for forty-eight months and found that 75 per cent had decreased angina. The rate of reinfarction seemed to be decreased by 50 per cent but life expectancy was less clearly affected.

DIRECT SURGICAL TECHNIQUES

Since the early 1960's direct revascularization techniques have been utilized. The earlier procedures included endarter-ectomy,[6] patch grafts[7] and gas endarterectomy. The follow-up examination for these localized procedures consisted simply of reopacification of the affected coronary artery, which usually was the right.

In recent years, surgical emphasis has focused upon com-plete bypass of the diseased segment of the coronary artery. One method entails anastomosing the internal mammary artery to the coronary artery distal to a severe stenosis. This technique was initially performed with a surgical microscope but is now done using the same surgical technique as for the vein bypass (see Fig. 110). Another more widely used method is the saphe-nous vein bypass.[8,9] Here one end of a reversed saphenous vein is attached to the ascending aorta and the other to the coronary artery distal to the atherosclerotic obstruction (see Fig. 111). In bypassing a right coronary obstruction, the vein is usually connected to the distal right or the posterior descend-ing coronary artery. On the left, the bypass is usually anasto-mosed to the distal anterior descending coronary artery. It is also possible to bypass the marginal artery, diagonal arteries or the circumflex coronary artery. Y-bypasses have also been constructed, having a single aortic ostium and two limbs at-tached to two different coronary arteries (see Figs. 112, 113, 114A, and 114B). This latter technique is being abandoned because of clotting of the limb in which there is less flow.

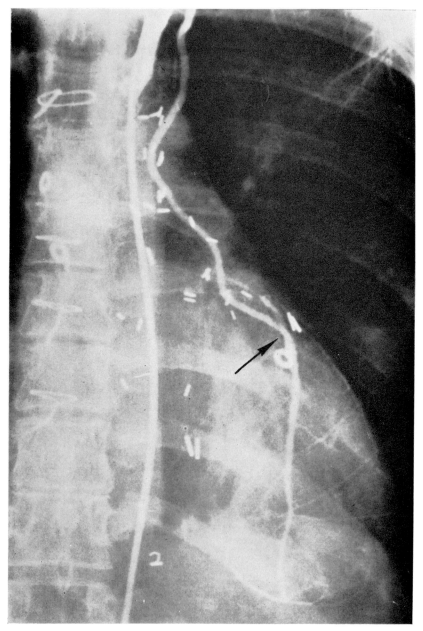

Figure 110. Selective left internal mammary arteriogram. Note that the mammary artery has been anastomosed to the left anterior descending coronary artery (arrow). Note the bidirectional opacification of the LAD.

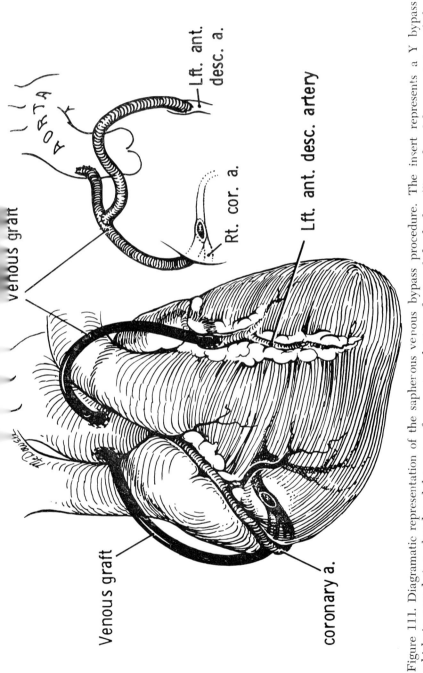

Figure 111. Diagramatic representation of the sapherous venous bypass procedure. The insert represents a Y bypass which is now being abandoned because of excessive clotting of one of the limbs. (Reproduced by permission of the *Am. J. Roentgenol.*, Vol. CX, No. 4, Dec. 1970 by Baltaxe, H.A., Carlson, R.G. and Lillehei, C.W.)

Catheterization of these veins can be performed as early as two weeks after surgery. Some even perform angiograms at the time of surgery using a C arm fluoroscope which fits under the operating table and they record the data on 70 mm films at 6 frames per second.* Most surgeons mark the ostium of

* Intraoperative 70 mm fluorography made by Philips Medical System, Inc.

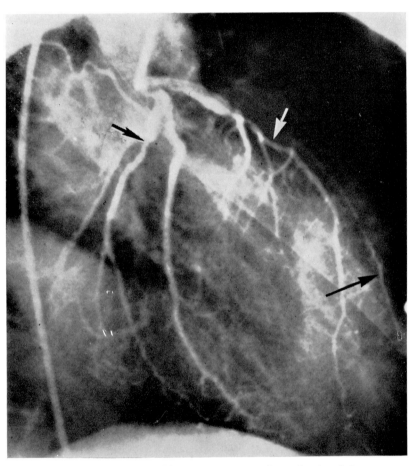

Figure 112. Right anterior oblique projection of a selective left coronary arteriogram. Note the complete obstruction of the left anterior descending coronary (short white arrow) and distal reconstitution of the LAD (black arrow). Short black arrow points to a stenosis of the circumflex.

the venous bypass by two metallic washers sutured on the adjacent aortic tissue above and below the anastomosis (see Fig. 115). This facilitates later selective catheterization. We have found the Amplatz right coronary catheter to be particularly suitable for vein grafts connecting the aorta and the distal right coronary artery. Catheterization of vein grafts from the ascending aorta to the distal left coronary artery often cannot be successfully performed with the same catheter because this vein first arches cephalad over the main pulmonary artery before turning down toward the anterior descending coronary artery (see Fig. 111). Thus, the catheter tip has to

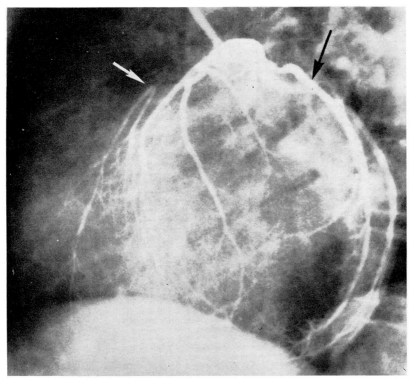

Figure 113. Left anterior oblique projection. Note the site of reconstitution of the LAD (white arrow). Narrowing of the circumflex is indicated by a black arrow but is obscured in this projection by overlying vessels.

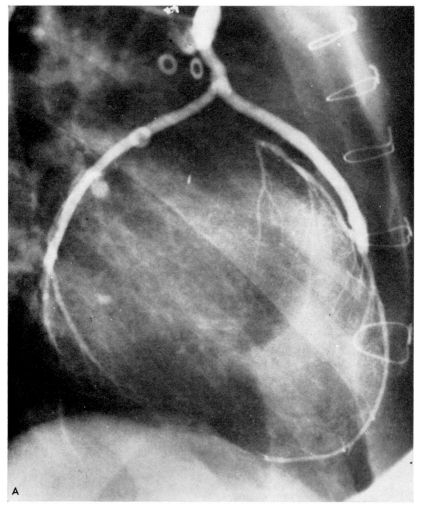

Figure 114A. Right anterior oblique projection of the same patient as in Figures 112 and 113 post-aorto coronary artery bypass.

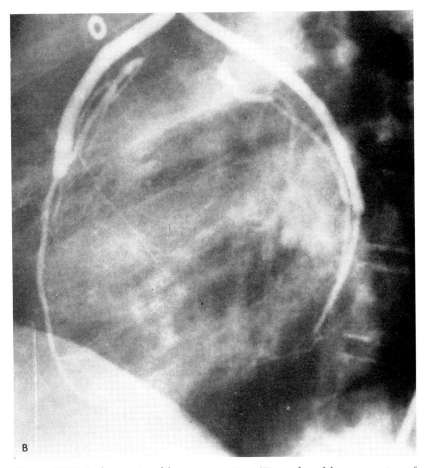

Figure 114B. Left anterior oblique projection. (Reproduced by permission of the *Am. J. Roentgenol.*, Vo. CXIII, No. 3, Nov. 1971 by D.C. Levin, *et al.*)

point cephalad in order to pass into the lumen of the vein (see Fig. 116). For the examination of these left coronary bypasses we have utilized the type 3 "Head Hunter" catheter which has been described by Hinck[10] and which is used primarily for studies of the brachiocephalic arteries.

Rapid serial radiographs and cine angiograms are taken during the opacification of these vessels. Both oblique projections are usually obtained on the lateral film changer, which results in a shorter object to film distance. The straight lateral projection is also useful when one studies bypasses of the left anterior descending artery. If the procedure has been completely successful, bidirectional flow occurs, resulting in filling of the entire arterial tree distal to the stenosis (see Fig. 117). If the procedure fails, the entire vein usually clots from the coronary artery anastomosis to the aortic anastomosis, leaving only a small pouch-like deformity at the aortic ostium (see Fig. 115). It is important to demonstrate this proximal remnant of the clotted bypass; otherwise one might erroneously suspect a bad result when in truth the angiographer failed to selectively catheterize the orifice of the bypass. Often a nonselective ascending aortogram does not opacify a patent venous bypass because of very slow flow within the vein.

When a bypass has clotted, we usually reopacify the coronary artery to which the vein has been connected, to determine whether the clot extends into the coronary artery itself. In addition to clotting of the venous bypass, other complications can occur. Reduction of flow within the vein may be due to intimal and medial hyperplasia (see Fig. 118). Clotting of the segment of coronary artery between the stenosis and the point of anastomosis of the vein has been noted on occasion (see Fig. 119A, B, and C). As a result of increased flow through the graft, collateral channels might cease to function (see Fig. 120A and B). In our material we have seen one case of a false aortic aneurysm developing at the point of anastomosis (see Fig. 121).

Effler *et al.*[11] have reviewed their results with the vein graft procedure. The patency rate in a study of two hundred patients was between 80 per cent and 85 per cent. In a later

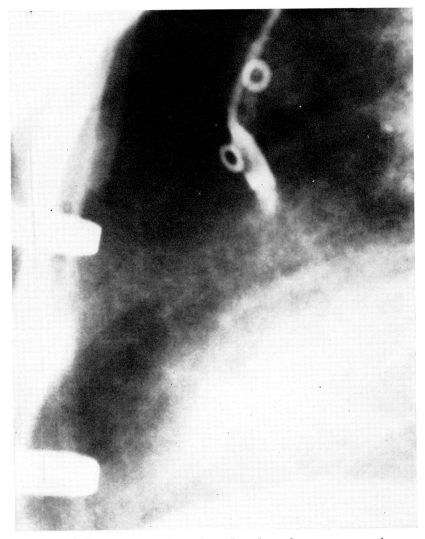

Figure 115. Lateral projection of a clotted saphenous venous bypass. Note the two metallic washers indicating the site of anastomosis of the vein to the aorta. When the vein clots, a small pouch-like deformity can usually be demonstrated. (Reproduced by permission of the *Am. J. Roentgenol.*, Vol. CX, No. 4 Dec. 1970 by Baltaxe, H.A. *et al.*)

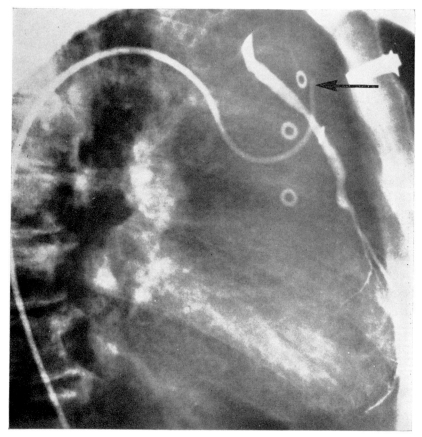

Figure 116. "Head Hunter" catheter introduced selectively into a vein-bypass connected to the anterior descending coronary artery. Note the cephalad position of the tip of the catheter (see arrow). Note the uni-directional flow of the contrast opacifying only the distal portion of the left anterior descending coronary artery. This finding presumably does not represent a completely satisfactory surgical result.

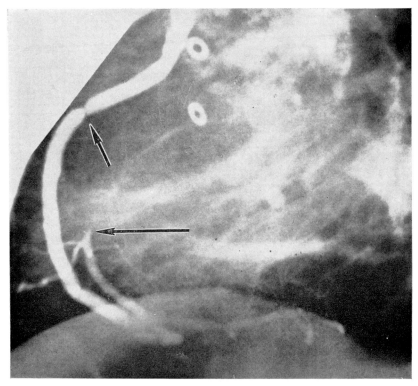

Figure 117. Left anterior oblique projection. Saphenous venous bypass from the aorta to the distal right coronary artery. Note the flow of contrast in both directions back to the point of significant stenosis indicated by the arrow. The short arrow points to a valve in the vein. The vein, however, has been reversed and therefore the flow of blood is not hindered by the valve. Some still question whether the presence of the valve may predispose to clotting.

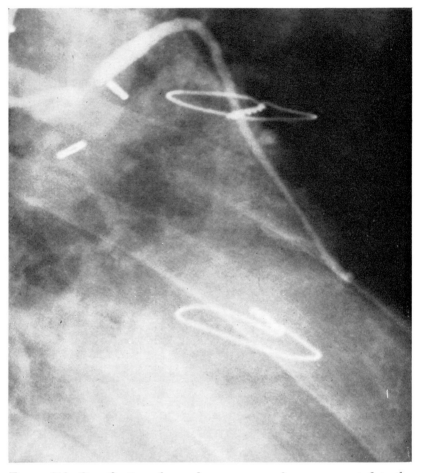

Figure 118. Opacification of a saphenous venous bypass connected to the anterior descending coronary artery. Note the diffuse and somewhat irregular outline of the vessel. The narrowing simulates an atherosclerotic change but is usually due to intimal and medial hyperplasia.

>>

Figure 119. A, Selective saphenous vein bypass angiogram. Graft bridges the aorta and the distal right coronary artery. Note the bidirectional flow opacifying distal (black arrow) and proximal (double black arrow) right coronary artery. (Reproduced by permission from *Radiologic Clinics of North America*, Vol. IX, Dec. 1971, H. Baltaxe)

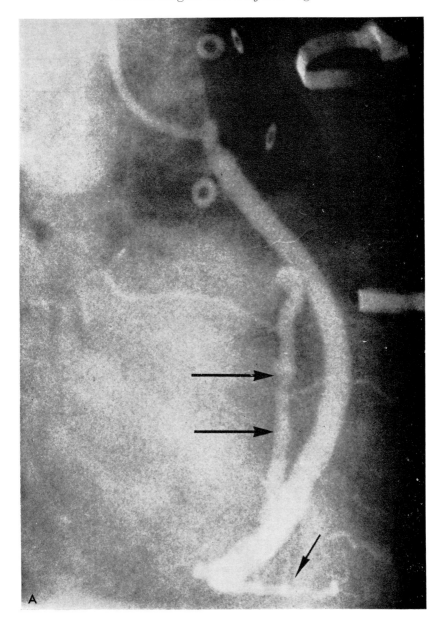

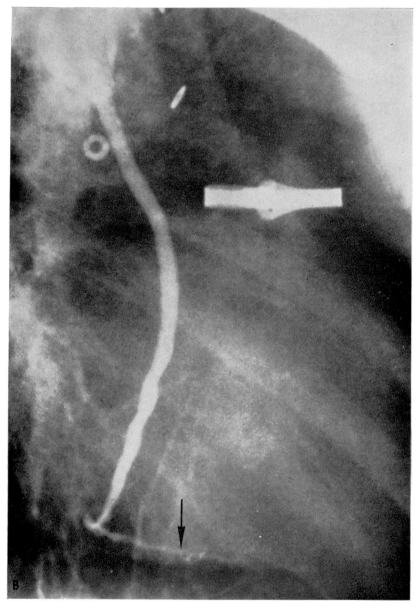

Figure 119. B, Restudy 12 months after previous examination. Note uni-directional flow. Only the distal right coronary artery is opacified (black arrow). (Reproduced by permission from *Radiologic Clinics of North America*, Vol. IX, Dec. 1971, H. Baltaxe.)

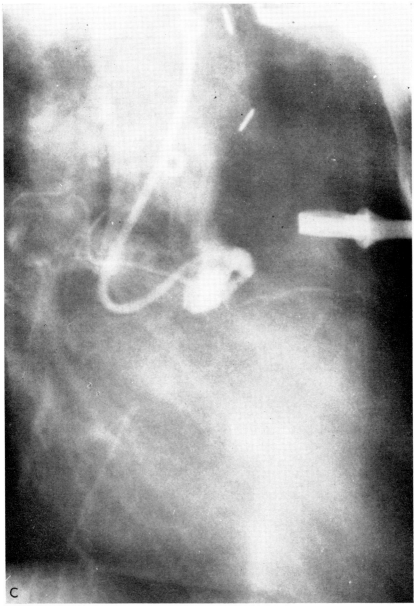

Figure 119. C, Selective right coronary arteriogram shows clotting of the right coronary artery from its origin to the site of anastomosis of the vein. (Reproduced by permission from *Radiologic Clinics of North America,* Vol. IX, Dec. 1971, H. Baltaxe.)

series of sixty patients operated upon in 1970, the same authors report a patency rate of 90 per cent to 95 per cent.

Patency of the graft seems to depend upon the quality of the vein, the type of runoff and of course surgical technique. The amount of flow through the vein is measured at the time of surgery with a flow meter and averages 70 cc/min/graft. If

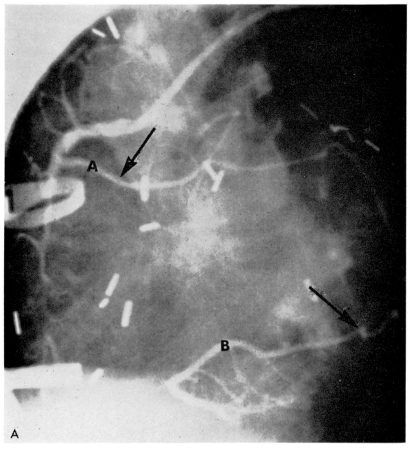

Figure 120. A, Selective right coronary arteriogram in the left anterior oblique projection. Note the almost complete obstruction of the right coronary artery. There is a large atrial anastomotic branch connecting (black arrows) the SA node artery (A) to the distal right coronary artery (B).

less than 40 cc/min/graft, graft occlusion is more likely. In addition, our own material indicates that patients with preoperative left ventricular ejection fractions less than 0.60 have a greater bypass failure rate.

Ventriculograms are always performed during reexamination of these patients to see if ventricular function has improved as a result of increased perfusion of the myocardium. It has been shown[12] that successful bypasses can restore normal contractility to areas of the left ventricle which previously were hypokinetic due to myocardial ischemia. However, once severe ventricular scarring has occurred, as manifested on the ventriculogram by dyskinesia, restoration of normal function is not possible.

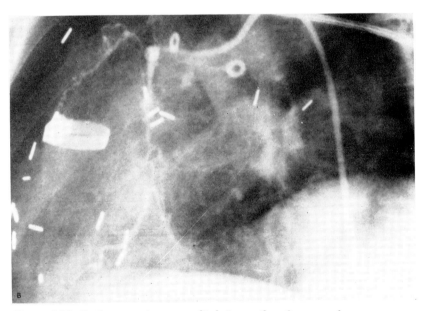

Figure 120. B, Same patient restudied 6 months after a saphenous venous bypass procedure from aorta to left anterior descending coronary artery (which is patent) and from aorta to distal right coronary artery (occluded). After occlusion of the bypass, a selective right coronary arteriogram demonstrates loss of the collateral branches.

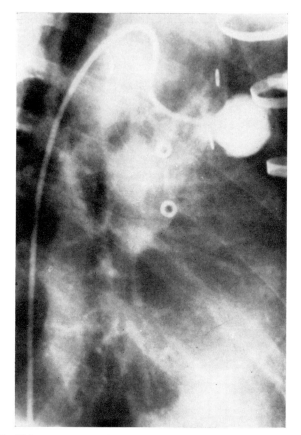

Figure 121. False aneurysm formation at the site of anastomosis between the aorta and the saphenous vein. Note that the vein is occluded. The patient was reoperated upon and a new vein was inserted.

During studies of the coronary bypasses, the same precautionary measures utilized in the course of coronary angiography must be taken. We have seen one instance of ventricular fibrillation during the injection of a Y-bypass.

REFERENCES

1. Vineberg, A.M.: Development of an anastomosis between the coronary vessels and a transplanted internal mammary artery. *Canad. Med. Assoc. J.*, 55:117, 1946.

2. Gorlin, R. and Taylor, W.J.: Myocardial revascularization with internal mammary artery implantation. *J.A.M.A., 207/5*:907–13, 1969.
3. Arner, I., Edholm, P., and Odman, P.: Percutaneous selective angiography of the internal mammary artery. *Acta Radiol., 51*:433–438, June 1959.
4. Dart, C.H., Jr., Scott, S.M., Takaro, T.: Transfemoral internal thoracic mammary arteriography. *Radiology, 93*:939, 1969.
5. Carlson, R.G., Edlich, R.F., Lande, A.J., Bonnabeau, R.C., Gans, H., and Lillehei, C.W.: A new concept for the rationale of the Vineberg operation for myocardial revascularization. *Surgery, 65/1:* 141–47, Jan. 1969.
6. Bailey, C.P., May, A., and Lemmon, W.M.: Survival after coronary endarterectomy in man. *J.A.M.A., 164*:641, 1957.
7. Effler, D.B.: Coronary endarterectomy with patch-graft reconstitution: Clinical experience with 34 cases. *Ann. Surg., 162*:590–601, 1965.
8. Favaloro, R.G.: Saphenous vein autograft replacement of severe segmental coronary artery occlusion: Operative technique. *Ann Thorac. Surg., 5*:334–39, 1968.
9. Johnson, W.D., Flemma, R.J., Lepley, D., Jr., and Ellison, E.H.: Extended treatment of severe coronary artery disease: Total surgical approach. *Ann. Surg., 170*:460–70, 1969.
10. Hinck, V.C., Judkins, M.P., and Paxton, H.D.: Simplified selective femerocerebral angiography. *Radiology, 89*:1048–52, 1967.
11. Effler, D.B., Favaloro, R.G., and Groves, L.K.: Myocardial revascularization. Cleveland Clinic experience. *J. Cardiovasc. Surg., 1*:1–8, Jan.-Feb. 1971.
12. Saltiel, J., Lespérance, J., Bourassa, M.G., Castongay, Y., Campeau, L., and Grondier, P.: Reversibility of left ventricular dysfunction following aorto coronary bypass grafts. *Am. J. Radiol., 110/4*:739–46, Dec. 1970.

CHAPTER X

PITFALLS OF CORONARY ANGIOGRAPHY

Angiographic artifacts or inadequate knowledge of the normal anatomy might result in the incorrect interpretation of a coronary angiogram which in turn can result in unnecessary surgery. Some of the most common pitfalls are given below.

SEPARATE ORIGIN OF THE CONUS ARTERY

It has been pointed out by Schlesinger and his colleagues that in approximately 60 per cent of patients, the conus artery has a separate orifice from the right sinus of Valsalva.[1] They called this artery the "third coronary artery." Usually, this orifice is rather small and is not entered during the course of selective coronary arteriography. Therefore, the conus artery is frequently not opacified, or else is opacified only by reflux of contrast from the orifice of the right coronary artery.

In some patients with left anterior descending artery occlusion, the conus artery serves as an important collateral pathway. Unless this artery is visualized, the existence of the collateral flow will be overlooked. A forceful hand injection of contrast with the catheter tip placed just above the right coronary cusp will generally fill even those conus branches which have a separate origin.

Other times, particularly when the conus artery is enlarged, the catheter may selectively enter with ease the orifice of this "third coronary artery." One must not mistakenly conclude that the opacification of the conus branch represents a main right coronary artery which is occluded distally. It is important to catheterize the right coronary artery properly in order to be able to evaluate the disease in this vessel.

210

SPASM OF THE CORONARY ARTERY SECONDARY TO THE CATHETER

Spasm caused by the catheter is well known to angiographers. We frequently see this in the renal arteries. The right coronary artery seems to be more subject to catheter spasm than the left. Whenever a narrowing is seen adjacent to the catheter tip in a major vessel, one must rule out the presence of spasm. Some workers recommend the routine use of nitroglycerin in order to avoid it.[2]

We do not follow this practice. However, whenever such a narrowing is seen either on the television fluoroscopy or the serial radiographs, nitroglycerin is administered and a repeat injection is made, not selectively into the coronary artery but rather into the corresponding sinus of Valsalva. The combination of the vasodilating drug and the nonselective injection will alleviate any catheter-induced spasm of the coronary arteries. Figure 122 shows a case of spasm relieved by nitroglycerin.

CONGENITALLY SMALL VESSELS

The anatomic variations have been discussed in previous chapters. The neophyte who is not familiar with these presentations might mistake a congenitally small vessel for a diseased one. Thus when the circumflex coronary is large, as seen in a dominant left pattern, the right coronary might be extremely small. Such a vessel should not be interpreted as being diseased (see Figs. 123 and 124). On the other hand, in cases of very large right coronary arteries, the circumflex coronary artery might be virtually absent.

MYOCARDIAL BRIDGING

The anterior descending coronary artery runs in the interventricular groove through the epicardial tissue. However in 1922, Ciranicinau[3] described a case of an anterior descending coronary artery which dipped into the underlying myocardium. Such myocardial bridging produces a transient narrowing of the anterior descending coronary artery when the myocardium contracts during systole.[4] This must not be mistaken for a constant finding and one should look at the appearance of the vessel during diastole at which time the flow through the coronary arteries is maximal (see Figs. 125 and 126). Bridging does not produce ischemia and represents a normal variation. It is important to identify bridging because an intramyocardial anterior descending coronary artery may be difficult to bypass with a saphenous vein. In actuality according to Favoloro,[5] intramyocardial anterior descending coronary arteries are much more common than is usually appreciated during coronary arteriography. Myocardial bridging seems to occur only in the anterior descending coronary artery.

SUPERSELECTIVE CATHETERIZATION OF BRANCHES OF THE LEFT CORONARY ARTERY

In a certain number of cases, the main left coronary is very short and divides almost immediately into left anterior descending and circumflex coronary artery. In those cases, it is possible

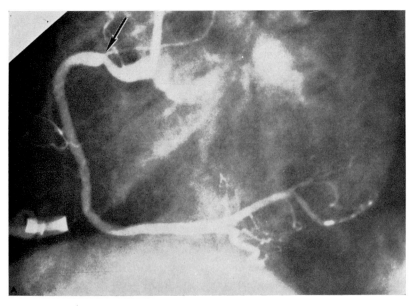

to selectively catheterize either vessel and to mistake the selective injection as showing an occulsion of the other vessel. Figure 127 demonstrates this point.

STENOSIS OF THE PROXIMAL PORTION OF A MAIN CORONARY ARTERY

The left main coronary artery is best seen in profile in a relatively shallow left anterior oblique projection. Since stenosis of

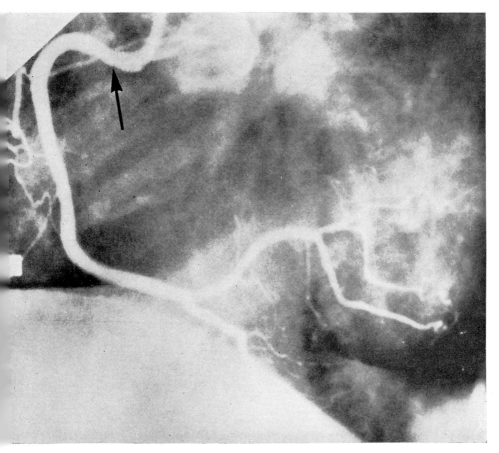

Figure 122. Left anterior oblique projection of a normal right coronary artery. A, Note spasm caused by the tip of the catheter (arrow). B, Spasm is relieved by nitroglycerin (arrow).

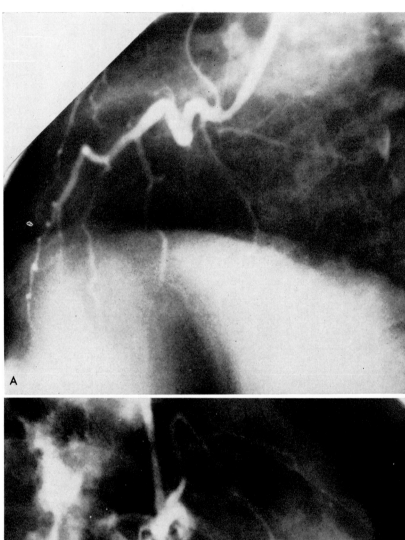

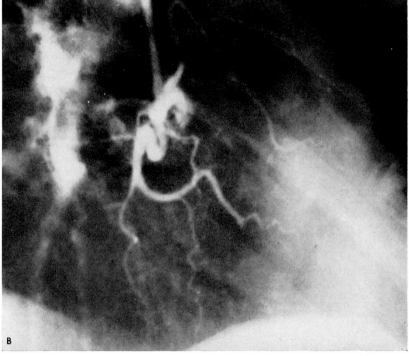

this vessel is probably the most dangerous of all coronary artery lesions, one must be sure this area is adequately visualized. It is possible to miss a stenosis of the orifice of the left main coronary artery if the catheter tip has passed beyond it (see Figs. 128 and 129). Generally, the hand injection of contrast material results in at least some reflux into the sinus of Valsalva, which in turn results in the visualization of the main orifice. Failure of reflux, together with a drop in pressure when the catheter is selectively inserted into the left coronary artery, may signify stenosis at or near the orifice. Again, an injection into the sinus of Valsalva might be necessary to properly evaluate this region.

The same applies to right coronary arteries which often present a stenosis at the orifice.

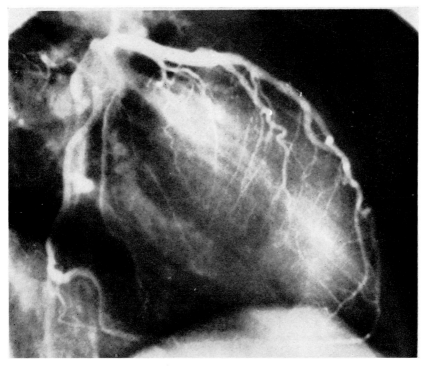

Figure 124. Selective left coronary arteriogram. Normal left coronary artery (same patient as Fig. 123). Note the large circumflex coronary artery giving rise to the posterior descending coronary artery.

≪

Figure 123. Normal right coronary artery in a dominant left pattern. A, Left anterior oblique projection. B, Right anterior oblique projection.

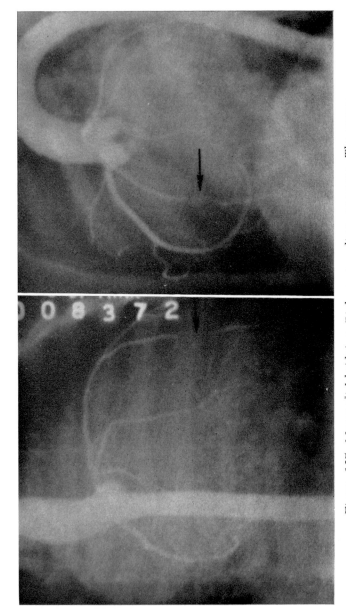

Figure 125. Myocardial bridging. Biplane ascending aortogram. The arrow points to an area of narrowing of the anterior descending coronary artery. These films were obtained during systole.

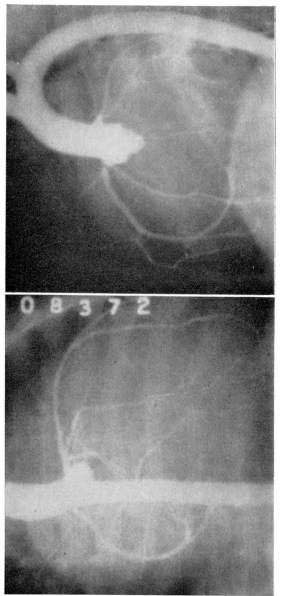

Figure 126. Same patient as in Figure 125. During diastole the narrowing disappears. (Reproduced by permission from Amplatz *et al.: Investigative Radiology,* Vol. 3, pp. 213–15, May–June 1968.

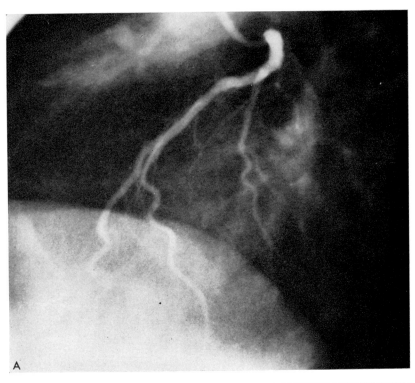

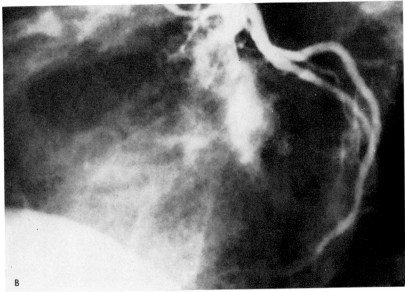

ECTOPIC CORONARY ARTERY OSTIA

On rare occasions, the right or left coronary artery may arise in an unusual position in its own or one of the other sinuses of Valsalva. In this case, searching with preshaped catheters may fail to locate the vessel. If either coronary ostium cannot be seen, and there is no other evidence to indicate obstruction of that vessel (such as collateral circulation or a ventricular aneurysm), the possibility of ectopic origin should be considered. Further searching with one or more catheters of different shapes should be carried out. If this fails, rapid pressure-injection of a large bolus of contrast into the aortic root will generally opacify the ectopic artery. This is discussed at further length in Chapter V.

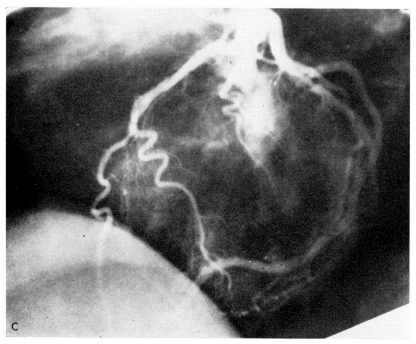

Figure 127. Superselective left coronary arteriogram. Left anterior oblique projection. A. Superselective arteriogram of the anterior descending coronary artery. B, Superselective arteriogram of the circumflex coronary artery. C, Injection into the main left coronary artery.

≪

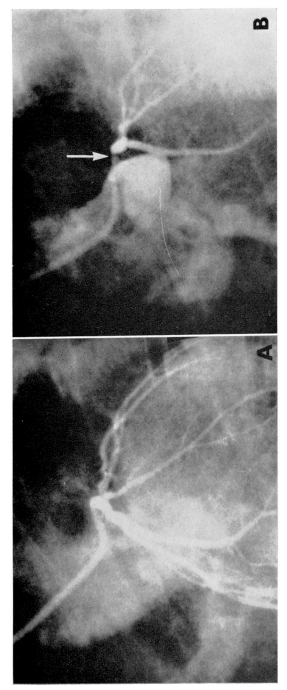

Figure 128. Stenosis of the main left coronary artery. Left anterior oblique projection. A, Catheter tip is beyond the narrowing and the lesion is missed. B, Injection of contrast into the left sinus. Note the area of severe stenosis (arrow).

FAILURE TO RECOGNIZE OCCLUSION OF THE
LEFT ANTERIOR DESCENDING ARTERY

In the right anterior oblique position, diagonal branches are often superimposed over the course of the left anterior descending artery from which they arise. Conversely, in the left anterior oblique position, septal branches are often superimposed over the course of the left anterior descending artery from which they also arise. It is therefore possible to miss a complete obstruction

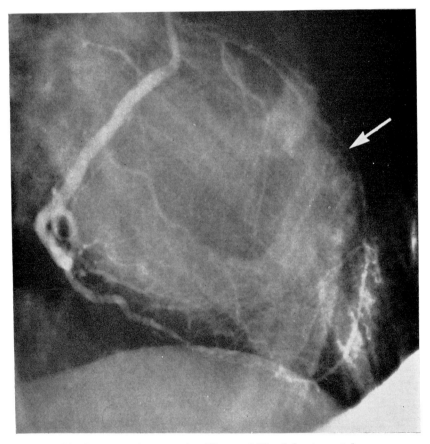

Figure 129. Same patient as in Figure 128. Selective right coronary arteriogram (right anterior oblique projection) resulting in the opacification of the LAD (arrow) through septal collaterals. This means that the lesion of the main left coronary artery is hemodynamically significant.

of this key vessel if careful scrutiny of the films is not made. One should keep in mind that a left anterior descending artery will always have septal branches and generally will pass all the way around the cardiac apex, whereas this usually does not hold true for diagonal branches (see Chap. IV).

MISTAKING A VEIN FOR A CORONARY ARTERY

When a coronary artery is obstructed, it may fill late via collateral circulation. By the time it opacifies, contrast material from other arteries may already have reached the veins. Therefore, it may be difficult to differentiate between a late-filling distal coronary artery segment and a cardiac vein. By carefully observing flow patterns, one can generally differentiate a vein from an artery, although the two may be close together.

REFERENCES

1. Schlesinger, M.J., Zoll, P.M., and Wessler, S.: The conus artery; a third coronary artery. *Am. Heart J.* 38:823, 1949.
2. Gensini, G.D., DiGiorgi, S., Murad-Netto, S., and Black, A.: Arteriographic demonstration of coronary artery spasm and its release after the use of a vasodilator in a case of angina pectoris and in the experimental animal. *Angiology,* 13:550–553, 1962.
3. Ciranicinau, A.: quoted by E. Geiringer: *Am. Heart J.,* 41:359, 1951.
4. Amplatz, K. and Anderson, R.: Angiographic appearance of myocardial bridging of the coronary artery. *Invest. Radiol.,* 3/3:213–15, May-June 1968.
5. Favoloro, R.G.: *Surgical Treatment of Coronary Arteriosclerosis.* Baltimore, The Williams and Wilkins Co., 1970.

AUTHOR INDEX

A

Abbott, M., 89, 117
Abrams, H., 8, 9, 16, 27, 41, 157, 184
Adams, D., 157, 184
Adams, F., 41
Amplatz, K., 16, 17, 23, 41, 42, 118, 121, 132, 195, 222
Anderson, C., 118
Anderson, R., 222
Anderson, W., 131
Annes, G., 131
Armer, R., 89, 118
Arner, I., 187, 208
Arnulf, G., 4, 8
Ashburn, W., 132
Austen, W., 131

B

Bailey, C., 209
Baltaxe, H., 42, 118, 131, 132
Baroldi, G., 86, 152, 185
Bellman, S., 5, 9
Bianchi, A., 86
Bilgutay, A., 7, 9
Bjork, K., 118
Bjork, L., 185
Bjork, V., 118
Black, A., 222
Boijsen, E., 42
Bonnabeau, R., 208
Bourassa, M., 41, 42, 185, 209
Bratt, G., 131
Braunwald, E., 42, 132
Bristow, J., 131
Brooks, H., 90, 118
Buchwald, H., 130, 132
Buckley, M., 131
Buonnano, C., 146, 157, 177, 185

C

Caldas, 3
Campeau, L., 42, 185, 209
Campion, B., 151
Caplan, L., 131
Carlson, R., 131, 208
Castaneda, A., 118
Castonguay, Y., 185, 209
Chacornac, R., 8
Ciranicinau, A., 211, 222
Cohnheim, 81
Coskey, R., 140
Curie, P., 118

D

Daber, K., 184
DaCosta, B., 155, 185
Dart, C., Jr., 131, 188, 208
Davis, G., 131
DeCarvalho, L., 8
DiGiorgi, S., 41, 141, 222
DiGuglielmo, L., 4, 8
Dodge, H., 185
Dos Santos, 3
Dotter, C., 4, 8
Driefus, S., 131
Dubiel, J., 42, 141

E

Eckstein, R., 148, 185
Edholm, P., 208
Edlich, R., 208
Edwards, J., 89, 107, 117, 118
Effler, D., 118, 197, 209
Ekmekci, A., 185
Eliot, R., 131
Elliot, L., 102, 103, 118
Ellison, E., 209

223

SUBJECT INDEX

A

Aberrant left coronary artery, 91
Acetylocholine, 5
Akinesia, 183
American College of Cardiology, 7
Amplatz catheter, 35, 41, 121, 195
Amplatz Technique, 17–24
Amyloid hyperplasia, 142
Anaphylactic shock, 125
Anastomotic circle, 62
Aneurysm
  false aortic, 197
  formation of false (*fig.*), 208
Angina, 36, 147, 177
  selective coronary angiography and, 126–128
  Vineberg procedure in relief of, 187
Angina pectoris, 147
Anterior descending coronary artery
  superselective left coronary arteriogram of (*fig.*), 218
  total occlusion of, right anterior oblique view of (*fig.*), 178
Aortic stenosis, 128, 129, 182
Aortogram
  ascending
    aberrant left coronary artery in (*fig.*), 91
    corrected transposition in (*fig.*), 111
    diagnosis of left coronary artery anomalies in, 89
    transposition of great vessels in (*fig.*), 105, 106, 109
  biplane ascending of myocardial bridging (*fig.*), 216, 217
  performed with venous pacemaker in right atrium (*fig.*), 7
Arrythmias, evaluation of in selective coronary angiography, 125–126 (*see*

also Selective coronary angiography, complications in)
Arteria anastomotica auricularis magna (*see* Kugel's artery)
Arterial insufficiency, 125
Arteriogram, coronary (*see* Coronary arteriogram)
Arteriography
  coronary (*see* Percutaneous selective coronary arteriography)
  transfemoral internal mammary, 188
Arteriotomy, 13
Arteritis, 142
Ascending aorta, frontal view of cast of (*fig.*), 44
Asystole, 123
Atherosclerosis, 35, 45, 50, 129, 130, 188 (*see also* Coronary atherosclerosis)
Atherosclerotic stenosis, 142–144
Atrial septal defect, left ventriculogram of (*fig.*), 63
Atropine, 5, 34
  intramuscular administration of, advantages of, 36

B

Bacteremia, 125
Bacterial endocarditis, 99, 107
  subacute, 142
Balloon catheter, 4
Bourassa catheter, 41
Brachial artery, thrombosis of, 13, 124–125
Bradyarrythmia, 123
Bradycardia, 36, 138